ANAESTHESIA AND PHARMACEUTICS

BOERHAAVE SERIES
FOR POSTGRADUATE
MEDICAL EDUCATION

PROCEEDINGS OF THE BOERHAAVE COURSES
ORGANIZED BY
THE FACULTY OF MEDICINE, UNIVERSITY OF LEIDEN
THE NETHERLANDS

ANAESTHESIA AND PHARMACEUTICS

EDITED BY

JOH. SPIERDIJK M.D. AND S.A. FELDMAN M.D.

with the assistance of Miss V. A. GOAT

LEIDEN UNIVERSITY PRESS

1972

SOLE DISTRIBUTOR FOR THE UNITED STATES OF AMERICA AND CANADA
THE WILLIAMS AND WILKINS COMPANY / BALTIMORE

Library of Congress Catalog Card Number 73- 188588
ISBN-13:978-94-010-2926-1   e-ISBN-13:978-94-010-2924-7
DOI: 10.1007/978-94-010-2924-7

Jacket design: E. Wijnans gvn

PREFACE

During the past twenty years there has been a rapid evolution in anaesthesia, so much so, that we stand on the brink of a major change in the role of the anaesthetist in medicine. Anaesthesia has now emerged from being a craft speciality, obsessed with details of techniques, to become a science concerned with the maintenance of life. As a result of our better understanding of the physiological and pharmacological effects of anaesthesia and surgery, new opportunities have been created for anaesthetists to apply their particular knowledge, not only to provide better and safer conditions for surgery, but also in resuscitation, ventilatory and circulatory support and in the treatment of chronic pain. This has resulted in the recognition of the anaesthetist as a physician specialising in applied physiology and clinical pharmacology.

The 1971 Boerhaave Course in Anaesthesia has deliberately tried to reflect this scientific basis of the speciality of anaesthesia by selecting for presentation in this book, subjects in which recent investigations have provoked new concepts and ideas.

We are most grateful to our colleagues who presented a paper and to the secretary-staffs of our departments of anaesthesia in Leiden and London.

Also thanks are extended to Mrs. Bongertman for the preparation of the proofs.

Department of Anaesthesiology   Johan Spierdijk
University Hospital, Leiden

Department of Anaesthetics   Stanley Feldman
Westminster Hospital, London

v

CONTENTS

Preface V
Contributors VIII

PART ONE
ANAESTHESIA AND THE HEART

Alpha and beta blockers in anaesthesia 3
H. LABORIT

Advantages and disadvantages of isoprenaline 18
M. THOMAS

Use and misuse of oxygen 24
G. ROLLY

The anaesthetic management of the surgical patient with a cardiac
pacemaker 30
P. J. JANSSEN

PART TWO
MUSCLE RELAXANTS

New concepts of the action of muscle relaxants 41
S. A. FELDMAN

The action of muscle relaxants of cholinergic mechanisms in the heart   48
V. A. GOAT

Changes of acid-base balance and muscle relaxants 64
J. F. CRUL and E. J. CRUL

The use of muscle relaxants in anephric patients 74
D. T. POPESCU

PART THREE
EFFECTS AND SIDE-EFFECTS OF ANAESTHETIC AGENTS

The truth about antihypertensive and anaesthetic drugs 91
L. STAMENKOVIC

Drug interactions in anaesthesia 104
E. L. NOACH

On the toxicity of halothane 116
B. R. SIMPSON, L. STRUNIN and B. WALTON

The dangers of anaesthetic agents to personnel working in operating
theatres. 130
JOH. SPIERDIJK

Index of subjects 141

CONTRIBUTORS

E. J. Crul, Department of Anaesthesiology, Sint Radboud Ziekenhuis, Nijmegen, The Netherlands.

J. F. Crul, Department of Anaesthesiology, Sint Radboud Ziekenhuis, Nijmegen, The Netherlands.

S. A. Feldman, Department of Anaesthetics, Westminster Hospital, London, U.K.

V. A. Goat, Department of Anaesthetics, Westminster Hospital, London, U.K.

P. J. Janssen, Department of Anaesthesiology, University Hospital, Leiden, The Netherlands.

H. Laborit, Laboratory of Eutonology, Hôpital Boucicaut, Paris, France.

E. L. Noach, Laboratory of Pharmacology, University of Leiden, The Netherlands.

D. T. Popescu, Department of Anaesthesiology, University Hospital, Leiden, The Netherlands.

G. Rolly, Department of Anaesthesiology, University Hospital, Gent, Belgium.

B. R. Simpson, Anaesthetic Unit, The London Hospital, London, U.K.

Joh. Spierdijk, Department of Anaesthesiology, University Hospital, Leiden, The Netherlands.

L. Stamenkovic, Department of Anaesthesiology, University Hospital, Leiden, The Netherlands.

L. Strunin, Anaesthetic Unit, The London Hospital, London, U.K.

M. Thomas, Cardiovascular Research Unit, Royal Postgraduate Medical School, London, U.K.

B. Walton, Anaesthetic Unit, The London Hospital, London, U.K.

PART ONE

ANAESTHESIA AND THE HEART

ALPHA AND BETA BLOCKERS IN ANAESTHESIA

H. LABORIT

To understand clearly the use of α and β blockers in anaesthesia, it is essential *firstly* to consider their action at the metabolic level of the cell.

This initial study will help to understand and explain their action on isolated organs, and finally their action on physiological and physiopathological processes.

It will then be possible to utilise these agents with maximum efficacy in everyday anaesthetic practice.

EFFECTS OF CATECHOLAMINES ON TISSUE METABOLISM

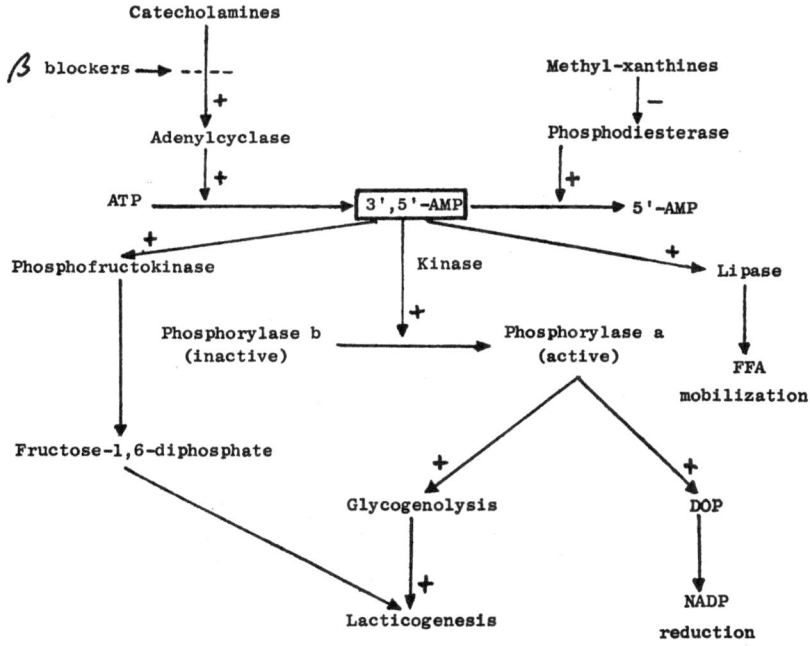

Fig. I

The metabolic effect of catecholamines is directly controlled by the increase they cause in the intracellular concentration of 3′, 5′-AMP or cyclic adenylate starting from ATP (1). 3′, 5′-AMP activates phosphorylase b kinase, which converts inactive phosphorylase b into active phosphorylase a which is responsible for the phosphorylation of glycogen into glucose-1-phosphate and, therefore, subsequently for the glucose-6-phosphate supply of metabolic pathways. 3′, 5′-AMP also activates phosphofructokinase, which is the key enzyme of glycolysis (2) and lipase, which mobilizes fats and causes an increase in serum free fatty acids (Fig. 1). Ahlquist (3) attributed the different physiological activities of catecholamines to their action on two different types of receptors, the α and β receptors. We have offered another hypothesis (4, 5) to explain this difference, and we based it on the differences in the enzymatic make-up and on the relative importance of metabolic pathway activity that exists among cells of different types.

Thus glucose-6-phosphate resulting from glycogen phosphorylation would be mainly utilized

a. either in the hexose-monophosphate shunt and glycolysis when the mitochondrial structures and oxidative processes are little developed (Type A);
b. or in glycolysis and the tricarboxylic cycle, if mitochondria are present in large numbers and oxidative processes are well developed (Type B);
c. or in either one of these metabolic pathways if both metabolic pathways are equally represented (Type C). The oxidation or reduction state of the NAD and NADP co-enzymes will then play a crucial role in the activation of the respective pathways that they control.

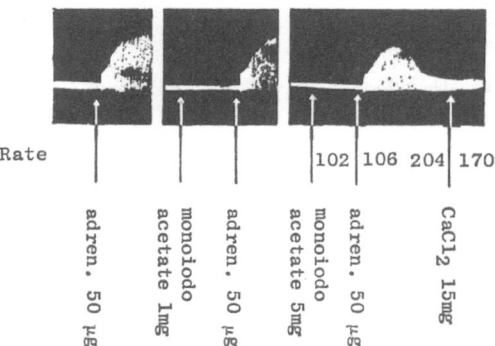

Rate   102 | 106 204 | 170

adren. 50 μg
monoiodo acetate 1mg
adren. 50 μg
monoiodo acetate 5mg
adren. 50 μg
CaCl₂ 15mg

Fig. 2. Rabbit atrium preparation. After an inhibitor of glycolysis (monoiodoacetate), the positive inotropic action of adrenaline is not blocked but it cannot be maintained.

At first it appeared that this hypothesis could account for all the pharmacological properties of catecholamines. Later, however, some authors (6, 7, 8, 9) showed that the conversion of phosphorylase b into phosphorylase a takes place after the inotropic effect of adrenaline, an effect that could not result, therefore, from an activation of the glycolytic pathway. Moreover, the positive inotropic effect of adrenaline is still maintained after administration of sodium monoiodoacetate or fluoride although for a short time only (Fig. 2).

It appears, therefore, that in addition to their action on the synthesis of $3',5'$-AMP with its known metabolic consequences, catecholamines probably exert a rapid effect at the membrane level which controls membrane permeability and calcium shifts (10). It must also be remembered that calcium activates directly phosphorylase b kinase located at the membrane level (11), and that calcium can counteract the inhibitory action of β blockers on the inotropic effect of adrenaline on the isolated rabbit atrium (12).

Since β but not α blockers inhibit the effect of catecholamines on the synthesis of $3',5'$-AMP, and consequently the conversion of phosphorylase a, the adrenergic α receptor could very well be an enzyme or a membrane component which would control ions shifts, particularly those of calcium (13). The penetration of calcium into the cytoplasm, leaving behind the triades of endoplasmic reticulum, would be the activating factor for myosine ATPase, and responsible for the inotropic effect of adrenaline. The synthesis of ATP, however, would be necessary for the re-integration of calcium into the membrane of the reticulum and for the maintenance of the inotropic effect. The addition of adrenaline to the perfusion fluid of an isolated heart preparation decreases cardiac glycogen and ATP content, and increases lactate produc-

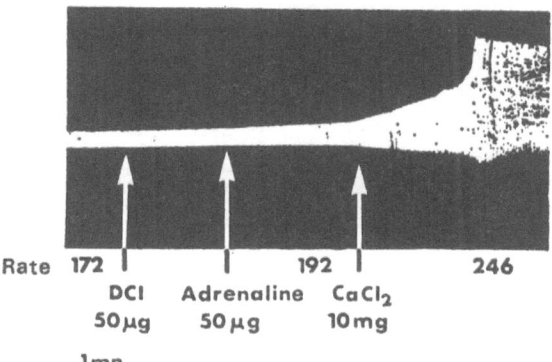

Rate 172   192   246
        DCI   Adrenaline CaCl₂
        50 μg   50 μg   10 mg

1 mn

Fig. 3. Rabbit atrium preparation. Limited inhibition of the positive inotropic action of adrenaline by a β blocker (DGI). Action of a Ca⁺⁺ salt.

tion. These effects are caused by the activation of glycogenolysis and of glycolysis. β Blockers inhibit these various metabolic actions, whereas α blockers probably inhibit the action of adrenaline on the membrane and on calcium shifts.

A. ACTION ON ISOLATED ORGANS

a. Action on the heart

Adrenaline causes an increase in contraction rate and amplitude in the isolated atrium or perfused isolated heart; these are the well known positive chronotropic and inotropic effects. These effects are inhibited by β blockers. α Blockers inhibit less markedly the inotropic effect, but leave untouched the chronotropic effect. Even with β blockers, the inhibitory effect is much more marked on the inotropic than on the chronotropic effect (Fig. 3).

The pacemaker and the conduction tissue correspond, in fact, to what we have called Type A. The chronotropic effect would then result from the speeded up repolarization of the pacemaker and of the conduction tissue due to the activation of the pentose pathway and glycolysis in this type of cell low in oxidative activity. Thus the membrane action of α blockers would not be able to counteract the metabolic effect of adrenaline on the specific tissue of the heart which is responsible for its chronotropic effect (Fig. 4).

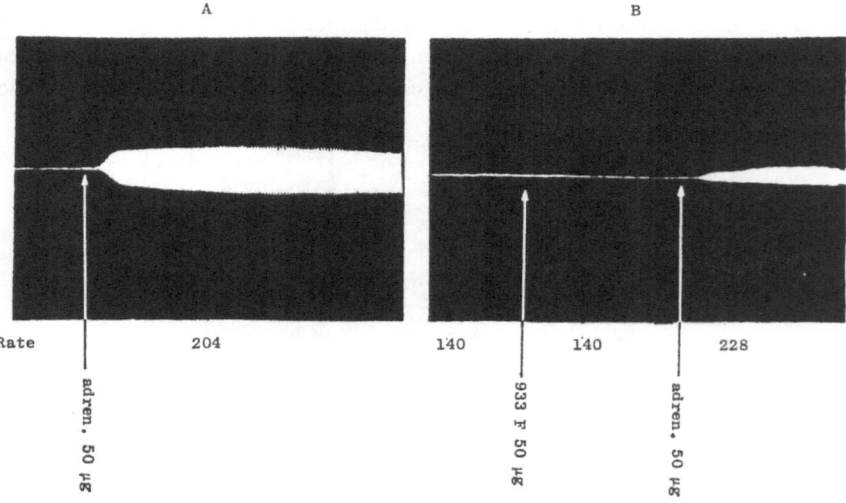

Fig. 4. Rabbit atrium preparation. An α blocker does not inhibit the positive inotropic action of adrenaline.

b. Action on vessels

The variations of vessel tone depend essentially on membrane phenomena and calcium shifts. Metabolic processes play a part only in the restoration of the initial tone (12, 14). β Blockers do not prevent the contracture caused by adrenaline and noradrenaline on isolated vessel sections (aorta, mesenteric artery, pulmonary artery) (Fig. 5), whereas the α blockers suppress it. In addition, a certain number of experimental observations lead us to believe that adrenaline opens up the arterial-venous anastomoses which belong to Type A (13).

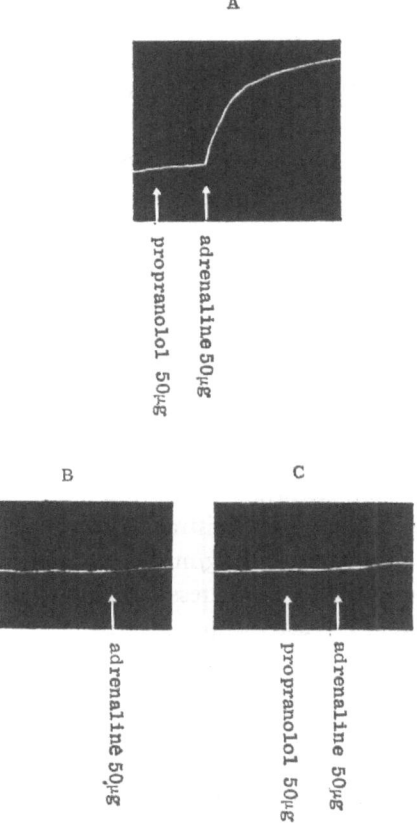

Fig. 5. Isolated rabbit pulmonary artery preparation. A. Bath with glucose: no action of propranolol, a β blocker, on adrenaline effect. B. and C. Bath without glucose (after 30 min.). Lack of effect of adrenaline.

B. ACTION ON THE WHOLE ANIMAL

In the rabbit, barbiturate anaesthesia (pentobarbital 30 mg/kg, i.v.) causes a
slight drop in arterial blood pressure (Fig. 6). This drop is not modified

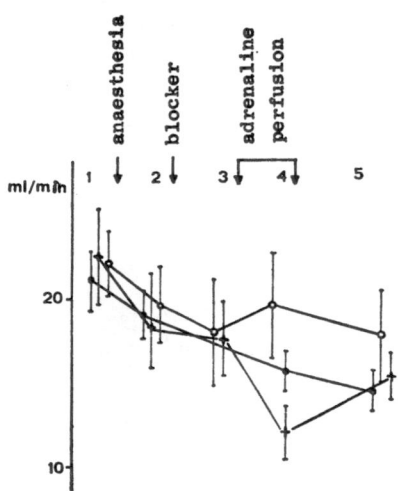

Fig. 6. Arterial blood pressure changes in an anaesthetized rabbit (nembutal) perfused
either with only an adrenaline solution (5 μg/kg/min.) (●—●—●); after the administration of an α blocker (933 F; o—o—o); or after administration of a β blocker (propranolol, +—+—+).

significantly by the administration of propranolol, a β blocker. On the
contrary, it is magnified by the administration of α blockers (933 F).

The perfusion of adrenaline (5 μ/kg/min.) for 30 minutes causes an initial
hypertensive peak followed by a progressive drop (tachyphylaxis). After the
perfusion is completed, the arterial pressure collapses to a level markedly
lower than the initial one.

If the adrenaline perfusion is combined with the administration of propranolol, a β blocker, the hypertensive peak becomes slightly more marked.
The progressive drop during the perfusion is much less apparent.

If it is combined with the administration of an α blocker, 933 F, the initial
peak barely reaches the pressure level observed with adrenaline alone before
the pressure drop caused by anaesthesia develops. The pressure, however,
remains stable during the perfusion, and after completion the fall is much
less marked.

In conclusion, therefore, in the anaesthetized animal, all the pressure variations induced by adrenaline perfusion are:

1. increased by β blockers,
2. dampened by α blockers.

DISCUSSION

The blood pressure drop caused by barbiturate anaesthesia is due to the decrease in cardiac output and to the systemic vasodilation, which results from a direct action of the anaesthetic on the muscle fibers of the cardio-vascular system (15).

α Blockers, which are without any action on the synthesis of $3',5'$-AMP (16), have little effect on cardiac contraction amplitude, but the decrease in vascular tone that they induce is a factor in cardiac output increase. On the isolated artery strip, however, α blockers alone have no hypotonic effect; they only counteract adrenaline induced hypotonia (17). The arterial hypotension that follows α blocker injection could perhaps be attributed either to

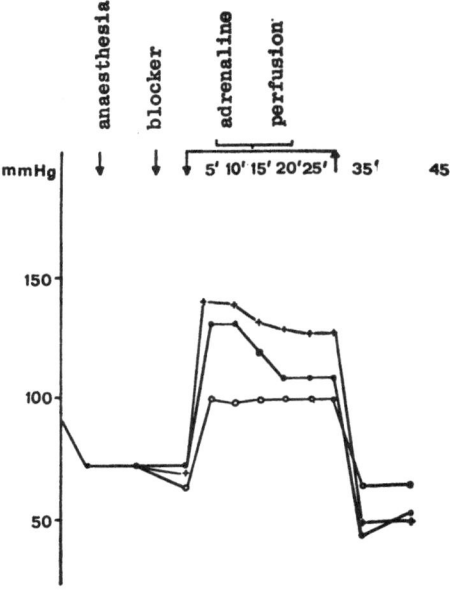

Fig. 7. Changes in mean oxygen consumption (in ml/min.) in the anaesthetised rabbit (nembutal) perfused with an adrenaline solution (5 μg/kg/min.) only (•—•—•); after an α blocker (933 F; o—o—o); or a β blocker (propranolol, +—+—+).

the opening up of the arterial-venous anastomoses, or to an antagonism to-ward physiologically circulating adrenaline. The residual hypertension during adrenaline perfusion results from an increase in cardiac output in the absence of peripheral vasoconstriction.

β Blockers inhibit the synthesis of 3',5'-AMP and the increase in cardiac output induced by adrenaline but do not inhibit the hypertonic effect of adrenaline on isolated artery strips (12). β Blockers have no action on Type A structures and, therefore, should not play any part in the opening of arterial-venous anastomoses. Thus the adrenaline hypertension facilitated by β blockers results from the increase in the peripheral vascular resistance and from a lack of compensatory reaction of the myocardium fiber. The blood pressure drop, which becomes more marked upon discontinuation of the perfusion, is the manifestation (a) of a drop in vascular resistance when vessels open up again to circulation, and (b) of an inability of the heart, under the effect of β blockers and barbiturates, to compensate with an output increase for the peripheral vascular resistance variations, whereas such a compensation remains possible under the effect of α blockers.

EFFECT ON METABOLISM

1. Effect on oxygen consumption

Barbiturate anaesthesia decreases oxygen consumption (18, 19) (Fig. 7) and this type of anaesthesia prevents the increase in cardiac output induced by adrenaline (15).

The injection of an α or β blocker does not significantly modify oxygen consumption. Adrenaline perfusion per se, under the same conditions, lowers it markedly, and even more markedly after a β blocker. On the contrary, following an α blocker, adrenaline increases oxygen consumption. During the secondary hypotensive phase, the decrease in oxygen consumption persists whether adrenaline is used alone or in combination with a β blocker. It remains stable after an α blocker.

Thus in isolated tissue slices or organs (heart) adrenaline increases oxygen consumption but decreases it in the whole organism whenever vasoconstriction is not prevented. β Blockers, which give a higher and more stable blood pressure during adrenaline perfusion, decrease oxygen consumption even more. This drop is really due to the fact that vasoconstriction maintains a hypoxic condition in certain tissue areas because β blockers, which decrease the metabolic effect and increase the vasoconstricting action of adrenaline, make thus more severe the drop in oxygen consumption, whereas α blockers bring back to normal the oxygen consumption increase due to adrenaline.

2. Variations in arterial-venous oxygen difference
Results are different in the conscious and anaesthetized animal.

a. In the conscious animal

Fig. 8 shows that adrenaline increases the difference in arterial-venous

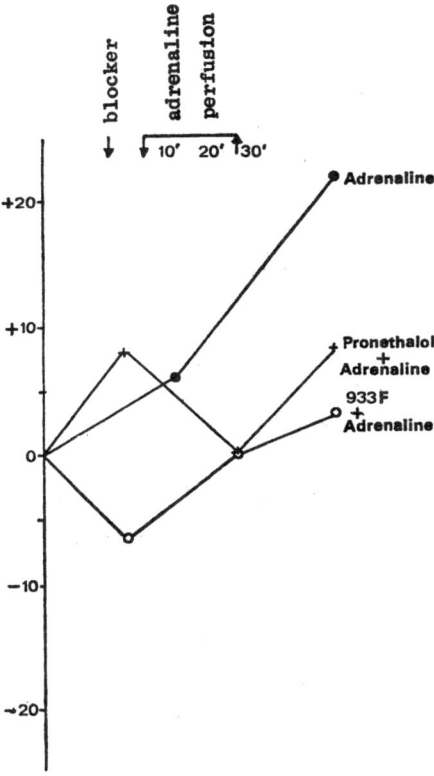

Fig. 8. Changes in the mean arterial-venous oxygen difference in percent of initial level in anaesthetized rabbits (pentobarbital, 30 mg/kg) and perfused with an adrenaline solution (5 µg/min.) alone (•—•) after the administration of an α inhibitor (933 F, (o—o); or of a β inhibitor (propranolol, +—+).

oxygen concentration (A-V DO_2). The same type of effect, although less marked, is observed when adrenaline is combined with a β blocker, probably on account of its antagonism toward the adrenaline induced increase in oxygen consumption. In spite of the opening of the arterial-venous anastomoses, the increase of the A-V DO_2 under the influence of adrenaline, combined or not with a β blocker in the conscious animal, must be attributed to the decrease in blood flow in the organs undergoing vasoconstriction. Indeed, α blockers cause a decrease in the A-V DO_2 that can be attributed to the combination of an increase in cardiac output and an increase in tissue blood flow.

b. In the animal anaesthetized with barbiturates, curarized and artificially ventilated
Fig. 9 shows that adrenaline has a tendency to decrease the A-V DO_2 and

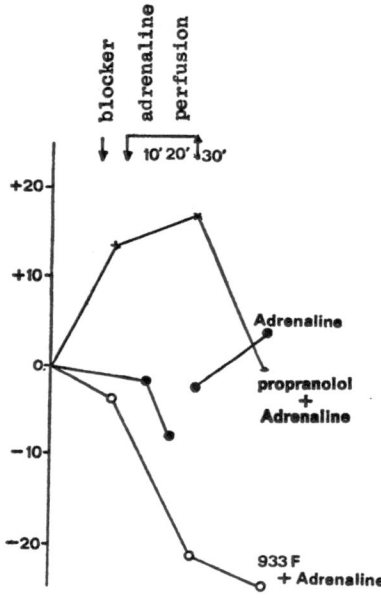

Fig. 9. Changes in the mean arterial-venous oxygen difference in percent of initial level in anaesthetized rabbits (pentobarbital, 30 mg/kg) and perfused with an adrenaline solution (5 μg/min.) alone (•—•) after the administration of an α inhibitor (933 F, o—o); or of a β inhibitor (propranolol, +—+).

this would appear to result from (a) a decrease in tissue oxygen consumption under the effect of the anaesthetic, and from (b) an increase in cardiac output. In this case, a β blocker increases considerably the A-V DO_2, and this can be explained apparently by a marked peripheral vascular stasis in spite of the decrease in tissue oxygen consumption. Conversely, an α blocker decreases considerably the A-V DO_2, and this probably results from an increase in perfusion rate and from the opening of the arterial-venous anastomoses. The maintenance of the inotropic effect and of the increased cardiac output, the absence of vasoconstriction and of blood flow decrease contribute also to the action of α blockers.

3. *Variations in lactacidemia*

Fig. 10 shows that the increase in lactacidemia is particularly marked after β blockers, and weak after α blockers. Since α blockers do not inhibit the

	Changes in lactic acid level at the end of the perfusion
Adrenaline (A) (5)	+ 14.8 ± 10.8 sd ± 5.43
933 F + adrenaline (B) (5)	+ 10 ± 8.83 sd ± 3.9
Propranolol + adrenaline (C) (5)	+ 21.2 ± 14.8 sd ± 6.6
	Between B and C (degree of freedom = 8) (t = 1.4) 0.20 > P > 0.10

Fig. 10. Changes in lactacidemia as compared to initial levels in the conscious animal (in ml/100 of serum).

action of adrenaline on $3',5'$-AMP synthesis, and on the activation of glycolysis, it is likely that lactic acid is reconverted into glycogen by the liver as fast as it is formed, since hepatic blood flow remains unchanged in the absence of vasoconstriction. If, however, the liver and splanchnic vasoconstriction becomes marked and stable, which is a typical effect of β blockers, hyperlactacidemia will increase accordingly. These results, therefore, stress very specially the significance of the hyperlactacidemia induced by adrenaline, and that its increase and persistance depend mainly on the hepatic and splanchnic vasoconstriction induced by adrenaline.

IN PHYSIOPATHOLOGY AND IN ANAESTHESIOLOGY

β Blockers mainly inhibit the metabolic effect of adrenaline, and α blockers mainly inhibit the membrane effects of calcium shifts. The action of β blockers, therefore, will be particularly felt at the level of the dynamic functions of the heart, and the action of α blockers will be felt at the level of the dynamic functions of the vessels.

In physiopathology, the sympathic-adrenergic reaction of various aggressions is controlled by the liberation of adrenaline (Fig. 11). The hepato-

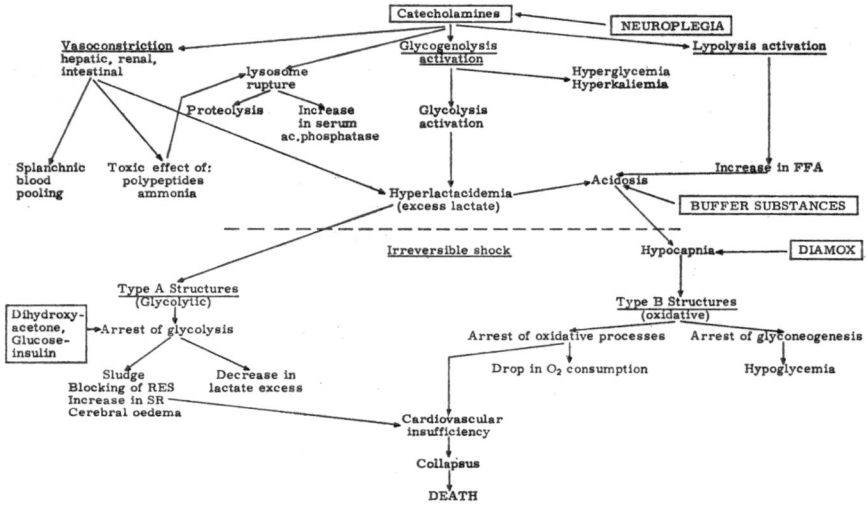

Fig. 11.

splanchnic vasoconstriction seems to be the basic factor in the lactic acidosis, in its persistance and aggravation. α Blockers prevent this vasoconstriction and its consequences, without, for that matter, depressing too much the dynamic functions of the heart. They will not be able to inhibit adrenaline-induced tachycardia, but they will not interfere with the stimulation of myocardial metabolism which is required to face cardiac output increase. A very fundamental point must be stressed: *Since α blockers inhibit the ability of the vascular bed to adapt to the volume of its contents, i.e., the blood mass, it is absolutely necessary, in case of hemorrhage, to control the blood mass by transfusions when α blockers are used; this we stressed as early as in 1952 (20).* If not, cardiac pump failure, cerebral anoxia and sudden collapse may result. If, however, the blood volume is carefully controlled, an α blocker will then maintain an effective blood flow pressure at the level of tissue; it will prevent tissue hypoxia and metabolic acidosis as well as the appearance of shock and its evolution toward irreversibility.

It could be feared that the peripheral vascular resistance caused by α blockers would dangerously lower coronary flow pressure in patients with coronary insufficiency. It seems, however, that the simultaneous decrease in myocardial work compensates favourably for this drawback, provided that the α blocker is administered progressively so that vasoplegia sets in as progressively as possible (21). There is no question, however, that under anaesthesia and in the pre- and post-operative periods the best emergency therapy for myocardial failure is 30 per cent hypertonic glucose and insulin, combined sometimes with a potassium salt; this is what we have called 'repolarizing therapy' (22).

To achieve an α blocking action, we prefer to use neuroplegics such as chlorpromazine or hydergine whose action is peripheral as well as central; this appears to offer more effective protection against the body's reaction to aggression (23). We prefer also to combine α blockers with an analgesic, and sometimes with an antihistamine (lytic cocktail) (24). Anaesthesia will thus be 'facilitated' and in extreme cases, surgery can be performed without anaesthesia (neuroleptanalgesia).

We consider that in anaesthesia much greater care must be exerted in the use of β blockers. We know that most anaesthetics used depress myocardial metabolism, including barbiturates. Combination with a drug that inhibits the utilisation of myocardial glycogen seems to be a dangerous practice, particularly since such a drug facilitates vasoconstriction and increases the cardiac load. Hjalmarson, Beviz and Isaksson (25) have stressed that hypoxia interfered with myocardial metabolism through two distinct mechanisms: (1) the liberation of catecholamines leading to an activation of $3',5'$-AMP synthesis which responds to β blockers; (2) a decrease in phosphocreatine and ATP content, as well as an increase in AMP and ADP which does not respond to β blockers.

As a consequence, the dynamic performance of the heart under hypoxia with or without propranolol remains definitely reduced.

The therapeutic indications suggested for the use of β blockers have been, up till now, mainly tachyarrhythmias. It is expected that they decrease cardiac rate and consequently the myocardial effort and oxygen consumption. Their inability to decrease mortality in myocardial infarct demonstrates, in our opinion, that the pentose pathway must be abundantly supplied to guarantee the healing of tissue lesions. It has also been suggested that they be used to prepare thyrotoxic patients for surgery since they decrease tachycardia. This indication seems more logical. In pheochromocytomas, they decrease cardiac excitability during surgery. But it is then necessary to combine them with an α blocker to avoid potentiation of the vasoconstriction response. Propranolol crosses the blood brain barrier, but we have never been able to show a clear central activity with cerebral stereotaxic methods.

Finally, although propranolol has been suggested in the treatment of arterial hypertension, we feel that it is contra-indicated in hypertensive patients scheduled to undergo surgery for the abovementioned reasons. The effect of a decrease in cardiac output and efficiency on a vascular system maintained hypertonic, seems to us a dangerous situation. A hyperactive heart in an anxious patient is essentially a case for tranquilizer or neuroplegic treatment for anxiety, whereas the effect of β blockers in anxiety has been until now without any clinical evidence.

REFERENCES

1. Sutherland, E. W. & Rall, T. W., The relation of adenosine 3', 5'- phosphate and phosphorylase to the actions of catecholamines and other hormones. *Pharmacol. Rev.* 12, 265 (1960).
2. Mansour, T. E., Studies on the heart phosphofructokinase: purification, inhibition and activation. *J. Biol. Chem.* 238, 2285 (1963).
3. Ahlquist, R. P., A study of adrenotropic receptors. *Amer. J. Physiol.* 153, 586 (1948).
4. Laborit, H., Mécanismes d'orientation des voies métaboliques en fonction de l'environnement et des agents pharmacologiques. *Agressologie* 2, 439 (1961).
5. Laborit, H., Structures métaboliques. Activités fonctionnelles et pharmacologie. *Agressologie* 3, 407 (1962).
6. Williamson, J. R. & Jamieson, D., Dissociation of the inotropic from the glycogenolytic effect of epinephrine in the isolated rat heart. *Nature (London)* 206, 4982, 364 (1965).
7. Axelsson, J., Bueding, E. & Bulbring, E., The inhibitory action of adrenalin on intestinal smooth muscle in relation to its action on phosphorylase activity. *J. Physiol. (London)* 156, 357 (1961).
8. Dhalla, N. S. & McLain, P. L., Studies on the relationship between phosphorylase activation and increase in cardiac function. *J. Pharmacol. Exp. Ther.* 155, 389 (1967).
9. Cheung, W. Y. & Williamson, J. R., Kinetics of cyclic adenosine monophosphate. Changes in rat heart following epinephrine administration. *Nature (London)* 207, 979 (1965).
10. Reuter, H., Action of adrenalin on cellular Ca exchange in guinea pig atria. *Arch. Exp. Path. Pharmak.* 251, 401 (1965).
11. Margreth, A., Catani, C. & Schiaffino, S., Isolation of microsome-bound phosphofructokinase from frog skeletal muscle and its inhibition by calcium ions. *Biochem. J.* 102, 35c (1967).
12. Laborit, H. & Weber, B., Essai d'interpretation métabolique du mécanisme d'action d'agents dits *beta* inhibiteurs adrénergiques (dichloroisoprotérénol, pronéthalol, propanolol). Etude expérimentale. *Agressologie* 8, 37 (1967a).
13. Laborit, H., Etude d'ensemble des mécanismes d'action de l'adrénaline et des agents dits alpha et beta lytiques sur le système cardiovasculaire. *Agressologie* 8, 487 (1967).
14. Laborit, H. & Weber, B., Etude pharmacologique comparée de la réponse à l'adrénaline de l'atrium et des segments d'aorte et d'artère pulmonaire isolés du lapin. *Agressologie* 8, 231 (1967b).
15. Karim, S. M. M., The mechanism of pressor action of adrenalin in pithed cat. *Brit. J. Pharmacol.* 27, 17 (1966).

16. Krishna, G., Hynie, S. & Brodie, B. B., Theophylline, a tool in the study of mechanisms of inhibition of lipolysis by adrenergic blocking agents. *Pharmacologist* 78, 87 (1960).

17. Laborit, H. & Brue, F., Essai d'interprétation métabolique de l'action de l'hexaméthonium, de l'hydergine, de l'yohimbine, du 933 F, de la chlorpromazine et de la caféine sur le segment d'artère et d'intestin isolés du lapin. *Agressologie* 3, 345 (1962).

18. Chance, B. & Hollunger, G., Inhibition of electron and energy transfer in mitochondria. I. Effects of amytal, thiopental, rotenone, progesterone and methylene glycol. *J. Biol. Chem.* 238, 418 (1963).

19. Lomax, P., The hypothermic effect of pentobarbital in the rat: Sites and mechanisms of action. *Brain Res.* 1, 296 (1966).

20. Laborit, H., La vasoplégie progressive dans la conduite de la transfusion au cours de déséquilibres vaso-moteurs post-agressifs. *Presse Méd.* 32, 693 (1952).

21. Broustet, P., Bricaud, H., Gazeau, J., Cabanieu, J., & Houtou, J. L., L'apport du traitement neuroplégique dans le traitement des infarctus du myocarde, de ses séquelles douloureuses et d'angor rebelles. *Presse méd.* 63, 1761 (1955).

22. Laborit, H., Intérêt majeur du glucose hypertonique en réanimation. *Presse méd.* 66, 444 (1958).

23. Laborit, H., Huguenard, P. & Alluaume, R., Un nouveau stabilisateur végétatif (1e 4560 R.P.). *Presse méd.* 60, 206 (1952).

24. Laborit, H., In: *L'anesthésie facilitée par les synergies médicamenteuses.* Paris 1951.

25. Hjalmarson, A., Beviz, A. & Isaksson, O., Metabolism of the heart with reference to beta blockade. In: *Inderal Symposium*, pp. 21-30, Copenhagen, 25-26 April 1969. *Int. J. Clin. Pharmacol.* supplement.

ADVANTAGES AND DISADVANTAGES OF
ISOPRENALINE

M. THOMAS

For more than ten years isoprenaline has been used in practical clinical therapeutics in a variety of circumstances. Its application depends upon two major pharmacological characteristics. First its chronotropic effect and its ability to arouse, accelerate and maintain natural and abnormal pacemaker activity (1) and second its inotropic property (2). Dose for dose, isoprenaline probably ranks as the most powerful inotropic agent available for clinical use. It is a pure beta-activator and as such is associated with peripheral vasodilatation as well as its dominant cardio-stimulatory properties. This becomes particularly relevant in its use in the various states of cardiovascular failure.

In the chronotropic context the use of the drug in practice is to accelerate an abnormally and pathologically low heart rate; bradycardia may be due to sinus bradycardia, and be associated also with first, second or third degree heart block. In each instance the essential fault in circulatory function is the fall in ventricular heart rate; each particular arrhythmia has its own variety of atrio-ventricular co-ordination defect, but the beneficial effect of isoprenaline in a chronotropic sense usually relates mainly to an increase in the rate of ventricular contraction. Such bradyarrhythmias are particularly seen after acute myocardial infarction (3, 4, 5), but also after cardiac surgery, and may occur spontaneously without clear evidence of major heart damage. The bradycardia hypotension syndrome (4), seen particularly in posterior myocardial infarction, is characterized by the patient having the general appearance of 'cardiogenic shock' with low blood pressure, pale sweating skin, and bradycardia. Sinus bradycardia is usually found but second degree heart block can also be responsible. Therapy limited to laying the patient flat and raising the legs is sometimes fully effective in increasing heart rate and improving cardiovascular function, but isoprenaline in a dose of approximately 0.05 mg intravenously can dramatically improve the situation by increase of heart rate and also force of heart muscle contraction. In the bradycardia

18

syndrome associated with second degree heart block isoprenaline is probably the drug of choice (6) if pharmacological intervention is clinically indicated, since atropine, although usually effective in cases of sinus bradycardia, is often less effective in second degree heart block.

In third degree heart block isoprenaline has been used both as a temporary and also as an on-going treatment over many days. By virtue of its ability to accelerate the rate of an idioventricular focus, and its inotropic stimulus, iso-prenaline can increase the ventricular rate to the point that the cardiac output is approximately the same as would be found in sinus rhythm at a comparable rate. Its use was extensively described by Vogel (1) and Zoll (7) some years ago, and it is still maintained by some that isoprenaline holds a major place in the management of acute heart block (8). Many centres, however, feel that the definitive therapy is the insertion of a transvenous pacemaker (9).

Paradoxically, isoprenaline can sometimes be used to eliminate foci of ventricular irritability when ectopic escape rhythms break into the long inter-beat interval in cases of bradycardia. Linanthal and Zoll 1963 (10), and Han and his colleagues in 1966 (11), have shown a very repeatable relationship between the incidence of ectopic beats and ectopic arrhythmias as compared with the basic rate of the ventricle. When heart rate falls to low levels ectopic foci are allowed the possibility to initiate repeated cycles and arrhythmias can sometimes become established. By increasing the basic rate of the heart isoprenaline can shorten the inter-beat interval such that premature ectopic beats are much less likely to become established. In such cases ectopic irri-tability can be eliminated by isoprenaline. Long-acting preparations of isoprenaline are sometimes very useful in the long-term management of such arrhythmias in patients with otherwise good heart function.

Positive inotropic stimulus of ventricular contraction is sometimes of value in cases of acute heart failure, as in myocardial infarction, and post-cardiac surgery. Isoprenaline is known to shorten the iso-volumetric phase preceding ejection (12), increase the rate of rise of left ventricular pressure for any given left ventricular end-diastolic pressure (13), increase the ejection fraction and the stroke-volume (14), and also to lower ventricular diastolic pressure. All these properties are in keeping with the powerful inotropic effect, and it has been shown in clinical heart disease in cases of chronic ischaemic heart disease, mitral stenosis, mixed mitral valve disease, mixed aortic disease, cardiomyopathies of various types, and also in normal sub-jects, that isoprenaline reduces left ventricular end-diastolic pressure and increases the cardiac output (15). The effect is less obvious in cases of severe aortic stenosis.

Because of the combined chronotropic, inotropic and vasodilation properties of isoprenaline, it is of great importance in the acute heart failure
situation. Since the peripheral vascular resistance changes little, or falls,
after isoprenaline the output load on the heart following the drug taking
effect is not as great as in the use of, for instance, noradrenaline which has
a peripheral constrictor property (16). With noradrenaline the blood pressure rises and the load on the heart increases, tending to exaggerate ventricular failure. With isoprenaline the peripheral resistance changes little and
the blood pressure effect is comparably less marked so that increased blood
flow rather than increased blood pressure is the dominant effect of the drug.

The veins often play a major role in syndromes of cardiovascular failure,
both as capacitative reservoirs and as a means of moving large volumes of
blood into the arterial system and lungs when venous tone increases. This
can have both advantageous and disadvantageous consequences; fortunately
increasing blood pressure, but unfortunately tending to exaggerate pulmonary oedema when left ventricular end-diastolic pressure is increased.
Consequently the effect of isoprenaline on venous tone is of great importance, and various pharmacological studies have been made to try to analyse
this as distinct from the effect of isoprenaline on other aspects of circulatory
function. While the situation is not entirely clear, it would seem that the
studies of Kaiser, Ross and Braunwald (17), using an extra-corporeally perfused canine preparation, are of particular note. They showed that isoprenaline always decreased the systemic venous blood volume, as judged by the
change in volume in a venous reservoir. This property was shared with
phenylepinephrine and norepinephrine. It was also shown that the systemic
venous bed contained both alpha and beta receptors, but in contrast with the
arterial bed stimulation of these two groups of receptors led to veno-con-
striction in both cases. Thus isoprenaline tends to displace blood from the
venous capacity system to other parts of the circulation.

Thirdly, it is self-evident that isoprenaline as a major beta stimulant can
be used to counteract excessive effects of beta-blockade. This may be important when patients on beta-blocking agents for angina control suffer
acute myocardial infarction when the heart failure in the presence of marked
beta-blockade may be particularly severe. In some instances it may be
necessary to override beta-blockade by isoprenaline infusion. Similarly
when beta-blocking agents have been used for arrhythmia control in cases of
refractory tachyarrhythmia, it may be that the residual beta-blockade is
profound and isoprenaline administration necessary.

In all these various situations familiarity with the use of the drug is necessary for optimal clinical management. Much of the bad reputation of isoprenaline as a potentially dangerous agent stems from excessive dosage in relation to the particular patient requirement. A general principle is that the smallest dose which is effective for the particular therapeutic object is the correct one. While a general statement of dosage, such as 0.05 mg intravenously for urgent use and an infusion of approximately 4 micrograms per minute for on-going intravenous infusion is of some value, it is exceedingly important to appreciate that there is a wide range of patients' susceptibility to isoprenaline, and giving a smaller preliminary dose often helps in assessing the particular responsiveness of a patient's situation. The onset of ventricular irritability and ventricular tachycardias often relates to the careless use of cheap plastic infusion apparatus. The controlling devices of plastic infusion sets are commonly prone to accidental displacement, with consequent major change in the infusion rate. With drugs such as isoprenaline this can be lethal. When it is contemplated that isoprenaline infusion may be undertaken for a period of hours or days the application of infusion pumps is to be preferred. At the same time, the patient needs close clinical supervision with monitoring and display of the electrocardiogram.

By virtue of the chronotropic and inotropic properties of isoprenaline an increase in the instrinsic contractile state and the external mechanical work of the myocardium always takes place (18). While this can be of little relevance in a normally healthy myocardium with good coronary vasculature and a potential of increasing coronary blood and oxygen supply in relation to the increased oxygen consumption, in some clinical situations the increased oxygen consumption inherent in the use of isoprenaline can be embarrassing to the myocardium. If coronary atherosclerosis is advanced to the degree that myocardial oxygen supply is compromised at rest, or is compromised when the consumption increases to any given level, then the inotropic effect of isoprenaline may lead to a relative hypoxia in the zones of poor blood perfusion with associated drop in intercellular pH, lactate discharge and failure in force of contraction. Necrosis may also occur (19). It is now known from experimental studies in animals that drugs such as isoprenaline also lead to an injury potential over those parts of the myocardium which are acutely ischaemic (20). S-T segment elevation can be profound following isoprenaline injection. These results are in keeping with the clinical observation that isoprenaline can sometimes initiate and perpetuate angina pectoris in patients with ischaemic heart disease.

In summary, the use of isoprenaline in practical clinical therapeutics is established in various bradycardia syndromes and is often very useful in situations of acute myocardial failure. The disadvantages are both practical and inherent.

The practical disadvantages are that dosage must be carefully controlled and the complications of excessive dosage stringently avoided. This entails the administration of very small doses in the initial assessment of the susceptibility of the particular patient situation to the drug, and the administration of the drug by reliable mechanical means when infusion is continued. Patients should be monitored by electrocardiographic display. The inherent disadvantages relate to the increased oxygen consumption which of necessity accompanies the chronotropic and inotropic effects of the drug. Care in controlling dosage will limit these to the minimum necessary for the therapeutic objective to be achieved.

REFERENCES

1. Vogel, J. H. K., Use of isoproterenol in the treatment of complete heart block complicating acute myocardial infarction. *Amer. J. Cardiol.* 7, 746 (1961).
2. Lands, A. M. & Howard, J. W., A comparative study of the effect of L-arterenol, epinephrine and isopropylartenerol on the heart. *J. Pharmacol. exp. Ther.* 106, 65 (1952).
3. James, T. N., Posterior myocardial infarction. *J. Michigan State Med. Soc.* 60, 1409 (1961).
4. Thomas, M. & Woodgate, D., Effect of atropine on bradycardia and hypotension in acute myocardial infarction. *Brit. Heart J.* 3, 28, 409 (1966).
5. Adgey, A. A., Geddes, J. S., Mulholland, H. C., Kecgan, D. A. J. & Pantridge, J. F., Incidence, significance and management of early bradyarrhythmia complicating acute myocardial infarction. *Lancet* 2, 1097 (1968).
6. Lown, B., Fakhro, A. M., Hood, W. B. & Thorn, G. W., The coronary care unit. *J. Amer. med. Ass.* 3, 119, 156 (1967).
7. Zoll, P. M., Linanthal, A. J., Gibson, W., Paul, M. H. & Norman, L. R., Intravenous drug therapy of Stokes-Adams disease. Effects of sympathomimeticamines on ventricular rhythmicity and atrio-ventricular conduction. *Circulation* 27, 325 (1963).
8. Hatle, L. & Rokseth, R., Conservative treatment of A-V block in acute myocardial infarction. Results in 105 consecutive patients. *Brit. Heart J.* 33, 595 (1971).
9. Furman, S., Fundamentals of cardiac pacing. *Amer. Heart J.* 73, 2, 261 (1967).
10. Linanthal, A. J. & Zoll, P. M., Prevention of ventricular tachycardia and fibrillation by intravenous isoproterenol and epinephrine. *Circulation* 27, 5 (1963).
11. Han, J., De Traglia, J., Millet, D. & Moe, G. J., Incidence of atopic beats as a function of the basic rate in the ventricle. *Amer. Heart J.* 72, 632 (1966).
12. Gleason, W. J. & Braunwald, E., Studies on the first derivative of the ventricular pulse in man. *J. clin. Invest.* 41, 80 (1962).
13. Reeves, T. J., Hefner, L. L., Jones, W. B., Coghlan, C., Prieto, G. & Carroll, J., The haemodynamic determinants of the rate of change of pressure in the left ventricle during isometric contraction. *Amer. Heart J.* 60, 745 (1960).
14. Dodge, H. P., Lord, J. D. & Sandler, H., Cardiovascular effects of isoproterenol in normal subjects and patients with congestive heart failure. *Amer. Heart J.* 60, 94 (1960).

15. Elliott, W. C. & Gorlin, R., Isoproterenol in the treatment of heart disease. *J. Amer. med. Ass.* 197, 315 (1966).
16. Sampson, J. J. & Hutchinson, J. C., Heart failure in myocardial infarction. *Progr. cardiovasc. Dis.* 10, 11 (1967).
17. Kaiser, G. A., Ross, J. Jr. & Braunwald, E., Alpha and beta adrenergic receptor mechanisms in the systemic venous bed. *J. Pharmacol. exp. Ther.* 144, 156 (1964).
18. Braunwald, E., Thirteenth Bowditch Lecture. The determinants of myocardial oxygen consumption. *Physiologist* 12, 65 (1969).
19. Niles, N. R., Zavin, J. D. & Norikado, R. N., Histochemical study of effects of hypoxia and isoproterenol on rat myocardium. *Amer. J. Cardiol.* 22, 381 (1968).
20. Maroko, P. R., Kjekshus, J. K., Sobel, B. E., Watanabe, T., Covell, J. W., Ross, J. & Braunwald, E., Factors influencing infarct size following experimental coronary artery occlusion. *Circulation* 43, 67 (1971).

USE AND MISUSE OF OXYGEN

G. ROLLY

Oxygen fulfills its metabolic role at the mitochondrial level (1). A stepward decrease of oxygen tension is found, going from inspired oxygen tension to mitochondrial tension. The inspired oxygen tension (150 mm of Hg, in normal circumstances when air is inspired) is therefore the highest value of a cascade fall of driving force of tension gradients to the cell mitochondria. Under pathological circumstances, various factors act at each stage of this cascade, to finally decrease the oxygen tension. It has been known for a long time, that in certain apparently 'normal' circumstances, during anaesthesia, post-anaesthetic recovery, following trauma, and other situations frequently encountered by anaesthetists, that adequate oxygenation may not occur whilst room air (20.93% O_2) is inspired. A supra normal oxygen concentration (30-40%) or even pure oxygen is sometimes necessary to raise the driving pressure at the beginning of the cascade, in order to supply enough oxygen to the cells of the body. The further down in the cascade that the lesion occurs, the higher the inspired oxygen tension and concentration required to treat the disturbance (2).

To understand the physiopathology of different situations, it is useful to consider the concept of oxygen availability. This concept was applied to anaesthesia by Freeman and Nunn (3), Nunn and Freeman (4). The oxygen flux or quantity of oxygen transferred in one minute is simply the product of cardiac output and arterial oxygen content.

Available oxygen/min. $= \dot{Q} \times$ arterial O_2 content
or Available oxygen/min. $= \dot{Q} \times$ (haemoglobin O_2 content $+$ plasma O_2 content)

or Available oxygen/min. $= \dfrac{\dot{Q} \times (1.39 \times Hb \times SaO_2 + 0.003 \times PaO_2)}{100}$

where: $\dot{Q} =$ cardiac output in ml/min.
$1.39 =$ oxygen capacity of haemoglobin in ml/g
$Hb =$ in g/100 ml of whole blood
$SaO_2 =$ percentage oxygen saturation of Hb in arterial blood
$0.003 =$ ml of O_2 dissolved in the plasma of 100 ml of whole blood/ mm Hg applied oxygen tension

24

PaO_2 = arterial oxygen tension in min. Hg

Under normal circumstances:

$$\text{Available oxygen/min.} = 5{,}000 \times \frac{(1.39 \times 14.5 \times \frac{97.5}{100} + 0.003 \times 100)}{100}$$

$$= 5{,}000 \times \frac{(19.7 + 0.3)}{100}$$

$$= 1{,}000 \text{ ml/min.}$$

Hence, the oxygen flux is determined by three variable factors: cardiac output, haemoglobin concentration and arterial oxygen saturation. It is important to note that the oxygen flux equals the product of these three variables (if we ignore the oxygen in physical solution), and that each can be reduced in certain clinical situations, particularly during anaesthesia and recovery from the same. At first this appears unimportant, since under certain circumstances all these variable factors can be reduced to say 2/3 of their normal value, without causing alarm to the anaesthetist. However, if prolonged for a certain length of time they may prove lethal. It is obvious that the safety margins are narrower than often thought, and during anaesthesia, and in the post anaesthetic period, these three important factors are often reduced.

Cardiac output is frequently decreased due to the direct depressant action of anaesthetics (halothane), and induced hypocapnia caused by hyperventilation (5, 6). The decrease may also be due to a reduction in venous return, as in the case of uncompensated hemorrhage, pre-operative shock due to hypovolaemia, and lastly, by sympathetic blockade induced by ganglion blocking agents, spinal and epidural anaesthesia, unaccompanied by concomitant volume increase of the dilated vascular bed. In the post-operative period these enumerated causes can all continue their depressant action. Post-operative shivering particularly attracts our attention. In this situation cardiac output remains within the normal range, but compared to the tremendously increased oxygen consumption, it is grossly inadequate (7).

The amount of haemoglobin can be low as in anaemia and hemorrhage. It can also be qualitatively deficient as carboxyhaemoglobin, methaemoglobin (congenital, or due to drugs such as nitrite ions and prilocaine), or be present as abnormal haemoglobin (foetal haemoglobin, etc.).

The arterial oxygen saturation can be lowered as the result of a decreased arterial oxygen tension (P_aO_2). This may be the result of a decrease in PAO_2 or by an increase of the alveolar-arterial oxygen gradient (A-aDO_2). PAO_2 can be decreased during anaesthesia due to frank hypoventilation, or accidental inhalation of a low percentage of oxygen. In the post-operative period the reduction may be due to hypoventilation, post hyperventilation hypoxia (8) or diffusion hypoxia (9). A-aDO$_2$ may be increased as a result of diffusion disorders, ventilation-perfusion ($\dot{V}A/\dot{Q}$) imbalance, or due to the existence of an increased shunt ($\dot{Q}$ s). Other contributing factors include age, position of the patient, type of intervention, type of controlled ventilation, deep breaths, Mendelsonns syndrome, post pump perfusion lung and pain.

The oxygen dissociation curve can be shifted to the left, with a decreased PaO$_2$ for the same arterial saturation resulting in impaired tissue oxygenation. This is seen in hypothermia, hypocapnia, carboxyhaemoglobinaemia, thalassaemia and under hyperbaric conditions. Recently attention has been drawn to a similar shift of the oxygen dissociation curve occurring in stored blood, due to a decrease in the level of 2.3 diphosphoglyceric acid (2.3 DPG).

It becomes apparent from the preceding summary of the possible causes of impaired oxygenation that the concentration of oxygen required (fractional concentration of oxygen in the inspired mixture FIO$_2$) is a function of the actual values of cardiac output, haemoglobin concentration, and the amount of shunted blood. The aim should be to obtain a PaO$_2$ of at least 80-100 mm Hg during anaesthesia, and although lower levels might be acceptable in the post-operative period, this would reduce the safety margin. An inspired oxygen concentration of 30% is sufficient to overcome gross maldistribution of ventilation against perfusion, in the presence of a normal haemoglobin concentration and normal cardiac output. However, 40% oxygen is necessary to compensate for a 10% shunt, and 70% oxygen for a shunt of 20%. An increase of oxygen concentration even to 100%, alone, is unable to compensate for a 50% shunt. Alveolar ventilation if increased, will, in itself, raise the PAO$_2$, whilst the inspired oxygen concentration remains constant. However, this effect will only compensate for a shunt of 5%, and is reversed in the presence of a more pronounced shunt, with a subsequent decrease in PaO$_2$. Pronounced hypoventilation can be successfully treated by increasing the inspired oxygen concentration from 21-30%. The role of oxygen consumption has received insufficient attention, for in certain circumstances such as post-operative shivering, it can be tremendously increased. Breathing air is only sufficient if alveolar ventilation is concomitantly increased.

It is clear that the oxygen concentration required varies widely according to both the clinical situation and the patient. In order to check the adequacy of the concentration of the inspired oxygen, important parameters must be measured especially the PaO_2. Because arterial blood sampling can only be performed intermittantly or in particular situations, we must often rely on trial and error. Since during most situations a moderate or pronounced A-a DO_2 is present, the PIO_2 (or FIO_2) has to be much higher than was previously accepted. To keep within the limits of safety, one normally errors on the high side, and frequently a high concentration, or even pure oxygen is given.

During the last few years, there has been a growing concern that pulmonary oxygen toxicity may result from the administration of a high concentration of oxygen. Many reports favour the existence of the toxic effects of oxygen (fall in vital capacity, decrease in pulmonary diffusion capacity, and development of absorption atelectasis). In chronic studies, capillary proliferation, hyaline membrane formation, alveolar wall thickening, hyperplasia of the alveolar lining cells, exudates, lung consolidation and interstitial oedema have all been described. However, evidence of a direct cause-and-effect relationship is not always provided, and several criticisms of the nature of most experimental as well as clinical studies, can be made. Humidification of the inspired oxygen is sometimes inadequate, and conclusions have been drawn from experiments using hyperbaric oxygenation, or from species that differ from man. In these studies the influence of maladjusted ventilation has often been ignored, as has the importance of concomitant factors, such as gastric aspiration, polypharmacy, underlying disease, etc.

The toxicity of high oxygen concentrations may be acting at different levels. A direct toxic effect on alveolar cells, capillaries and surface lining of the alveoli is possible. Rapid absorption of oxygen in the absence of nitrogen is probable if airway closure or obstruction is present (10, 11). Impairment of mucociliary transport has been described (12, 13). The high partial pressures of oxygen can act indirectly on the control of ventilation and on the adequacy of gaseous exchange, when the ventilatory response to carbon dioxide is impaired. This occurs in patients with chronic respiratory insufficiency. The particular toxicity of oxygen in the neonate, causing retrolental fibroplasia, is well documented.

Winter et al. (14) suggested that in the presence of high alveolar oxygen tensions, a low or normal arterial oxygen tension may partially protect from the pulmonary toxicity of oxygen. This, however, has not been confirmed by Miller et al. (15), who used a different approach to this problem. In a clinical study, Singer et al. (16) demonstrated no significant difference in shunt, compliance, VD/VT ratio, or clinical course after open-heart surgery, in two groups of patients who received either 100% O_2 or 42% O_2 (PaO_2 80-120 min. Hg) during a 24 hour period.

On a practical basis it is possible to summarise the current thinkings about oxygen administration as follows. During anaesthesia, oxygen should be liberally administered as necessary, this means 50% for higher abdominal surgery (17) and even more than 50% for thoracic, according to Hallowell (18). This short term administration of oxygen, coupled with adequate humidification (semi-closed circuit, heated water or ultrasonic humidifier) is not deleterious to the patient and provides additional safety during cardiovascular disturbances, especially during cardiac surgery. In the post-operative period, short term administration of oxygen should be done with low concentrations (FIO_2 = 30-40%) to combat ventilation-perfusion disturbances. If a higher concentration or prolonged administration is necessary, and this is especially so in cases requiring controlled ventilation, regular arterial measurements should be carried out, in order to administer the least possible oxygen concentration, compatible with a PaO_2 around 80-100 mm Hg. In this way, the administration of high oxygen concentrations, or even pure oxygen, or hyperbaric oxygen, can be safe within certain limits. However, it becomes most certainly unsafe when the administration of oxygen is uncontrolled.

REFERENCES

1. Leigh, J. M., Oxygen therapy at ambient pressure. In: Scurr and Feldman, *Scientific foundations of anaesthesia*. p. 200. London 1970.
2. Campbell, E. J. M., Methods of oxygen administration in respiratory failure. *Ann. N.Y. Acad. Sci.* 22, 221 (1965).
3. Freeman, J. & Nunn, J. F., Ventilation-perfusion relationships after haemorrhage. *Clin. Sci.* 24, 135 (1963).
4. Nunn, J. F. & Freeman, J., Problems of oxygenation and oxygen transport in anaesthesia. *Anaesthesia* 19, 120 (1964).
5. Prys-Roberts, C., Kelman, G. R., Greenbaum, R. & Robinson, R. H., Circulatory influences of artificial ventilation during nitrous oxide anaesthesia in man. II. Results: The relative influence of mean intrathoracic pressure and arterial carbon dioxide tension. *Brit. J. Anaesth.* 39, 533 (1967).
6. Prys-Roberts, C., Kelman, G. R., Greenbaum, R., Kain, M. L. & Bay, J., Hemodynamics and alveolar-arterial PO_2 differences at varying Pa_{CO_2} in anaesthetised man. *J. appl. Physiol.* 25, 80 (1968).
7. Bay, J., Nunn, J. F. & Prys-Roberts, C., Factors influencing arterial PO_2 during recovery from anaesthesia. *Brit. J. Anaesth.* 40, 398 (1968).
8. Sullivan, S. F., Patterson, R. W. & Papper, E. M., Posthyperventilation hypoxia. *J. appl. Physiol.* 22, 431 (1967).
9. Fink, B. R., Diffusion anoxia (in recovery from anaesthesia). *Anesthesiology* 16, 511-519, (1955).

10. Dale, W. A. & Rahn, H., Rate of gas absorption during atelectasis. *Amer. J. Physio..* 170, 606 (1952).
11. Rahn, H. & Farhi, L., Gaseous environment and atelectasis. *Fed. Proc.* 22, 1035 (1963).
12. Laurenzi, G. A., Yin, S. & Guarneri, J. J., Adverse effect of oxygen on tracheal mucus flow. *New Engl. J. Med.* 279, 333 (1968).
13. Marin, M. G. & Morrow, P. E. Effect of changing inspired O_2 and CO_2 levels on tracheal mucociliary transport rate. *J. appl. Physiol.* 27, 385 (1969).
14. Winter, P. M., Gupta, R. K., Michalski, A. H. & Lanphier, E. H., Modification of hyperbaric oxygen toxicity of experimental venous admixture. *J. appl. Physiol.* 23, 954 (1967).
15. Miller, W. W., Waldhausen, J. A. & Rashkind, W. J., Comparison of oxygen poisoning of the lung in cyanotic and acyanotic dogs. *New Engl. J. Med.* 282, 943 (1970).
16. Singer, M. M., Wright, F., Stanley, L. L., Roe, B. B. & Hamilton, W. K., Oxygen toxicity in man: a prospective study in patients after open-heart surgery. *New Engl. J. Med.* 283, 1473 (1970).
17. Slater, E. M., Nilson, S. E., Leake, D. L., Parry, W. L., Laver, M. B., Hedley-Whyte, J. & Bendixen, H. H., Arterial oxygen tension measurements during nitrous oxide-oxygen anesthesia. *Anesthesiology* 26, 642 (1965).
18. Hallowell, P., Hedley-Whyte, J., Austen, W. G. & Laver, M. B., Oxygenation during closed mitral valvulotomy with halothane and nitrous oxide anesthesia. *Anesthesiology* 26, 248-249 (1965).

THE ANAESTHETIC MANAGEMENT OF THE SURGICAL
PATIENT WITH A CARDIAC PACEMAKER

P. J. JANSSEN

Each year an estimated number of 50-60 cardiac pacemakers are implanted per 1 million population in the Western European countries (1). In Holland during 1970 their number was approximately 900. The patients fitted with a pacemaker usually do not fall into the category of 'otherwise young healthy individuals'. Being older they often suffer from other diseases, which sometimes requires surgical intervention. If they are young they will, with the help of their pacemaker, grow older and then come into the same 'old category'.

If surgery is indicated, it is in general the anaesthetic management which will determine the final outcome of the intervention.

It is not our intention to deal in this paper with the anaesthetic management of the patient who is to have a cardiac pacemaker implanted, but rather to discuss anaesthesia for patients already fitted with a pacemaker.

It is outside the scope of this presentation to discuss the cardiological indications for temporary or permanent cardiac pacing.

Nor will the various types of pacemakers and their principles be discussed. It should, however, be remembered that two basic systems of pacing are used: these are the bipolar, in which both anode and cathode are in or on the heart; and the unipolar, in which only one pole (usually the cathode) is in contact with the heart, the other pole being situated elsewhere in the body (usually in the pacemaker body itself). Before discussing the specific anaesthetic problems, a few technical and mechanical problems are dealt with first.

A. TECHNICAL AND MECHANICAL PROBLEMS

1. Pacemaker failure may result from technical faults within the pacemaker, or from exhaustion of the batteries.

2. Failure to pace may also result from problems with electrodes:

30

a. They may be broken; sometimes there is intermittent pacing with changes in body position, when the inner metal core of the electrode is completely broken, whilst the outer protective sheath remains intact.

b. The tip of the stimulating electrode in (or on) the heart may have become dislodged. Usually the tip of the intravenous electrode is firmly fixed in place in the right ventricle, two to three days after implantation.

c. Wherever the battery is implanted, the surgeon should remember that electrodes are running from it to the heart; his incision and dissection should not disrupt them!

d. With abnormal body positions great care should be taken (lateral decubitus, extreme jack knife, even too high leg supports). They might cause kinking and/or breaking of the electrodes, or these might be pulled out of their connections with the battery.

3. The proper functioning of the pacemaker should always be checked pre-operatively by a cardiologist who is qualified in this respect. The type and working principle of the apparatus should be known. If these facilities are not available in the hospital, then the patient should be referred for surgery and anaesthesia to a centre which is well equipped for these procedures.

4. Elevation of the stimulus threshold usually occurs during the first month after implantation of a cardiac pacemaker. A change in this threshold might also occur after direct trauma to the abdomen or chest. Parasympathetic stimulation increases, adrenergic stimulation decreases this threshold, and therefore makes the heart more irritable.

B. SPECIFIC ANAESTHETIC PROBLEMS

1. a. Premedication

In order to keep the airways free of secretions, atropine is always indicated. Atropine will naturally not influence the heart rate in these patients, but it will exert all its other parasympatholytic influences on the various organ systems. Optimal sedation is essential. An anxious patient will have an increase in circulating catecholamines; this will increase the risk of ventricular extra-systoles and ventricular fibrillation. A too heavily sedated patient will suffer from the results of impaired regulation of blood pressure and blood flow (diminished venous return after peripheral vasoldilatation). Of the various premedicants used the most preferable seem to be promethazine

(Phenergan) in a dosage of 0.5 mg/kg i.m., or diazepam (Valium) in a dosage of 0.1 mg/kg intramuscularly, which has even less effect on the circulation.

b. It would seem almost unnecessary to emphasize, that in the pre-operative period the patient should be in a quiet environment. Induction of anaesthesia should be done in a quiet atmosphere, where simple but all-important human attention should be paid to this person seeking our help.

c. The explanation to the patient, concerning the various precautionary measures taken, will prevent the occurrence of unnecessary fears (catecholamines!). The patient will then more easily accept the following measures instituted prior to induction of anaesthesia:

i. A standard four lead electrocardiogram is set up; this should be constantly visible on an electrocardioscope; abnormalities should preferably be recorded automatically.

ii. In a patient with a cardiac pacemaker we are not so interested in the electrical activity of the heart, but rather in the mechanical activity of the ventricular myocardium. This is best reflected in the peripheral pulse wave. It is therefore essential to use a plethysmoscope, with the possibility of a graphical recording, the pickup of which is attached to a fingertip or ear lobe.

iii. Whilst these preparations are being made it is wise to pre-oxygenate the patient. A well oxygenated substrate is less prone to other noxious influences on the one hand, and on the other hand has more 'natural buffer' in case of calamities during induction.

iv. A short wide-bore intravenous canula should be in place before anaesthesia starts.

v. Absolute hypovolemia should be restored to normal, prior to induction, as should a relative hypovolemia, preferably with relatively short acting plasma volume expanders (low molecular dextrans). It is in this respect important to realise that some of these fluids (especially Haemaccel) contain relatively large quantities of calcium, and should therefore not be used in these circumstances. A useful tool in assessing the 'volemia' is the central venous pressure.

d. Naturally the anaesthetist responsible for the anaesthesia, should be thoroughly familiar with the patient he has to protect. He should know the technical characteristics of the pacemaker, and also be informed about cardio-vascular and respiratory functions of the patient. Recent electrolyte values (K, Ca) should be available. He should have a reasonable impression about the patient's 'volemia'.

2. Is general anaesthesia indicated?

The necessity of general anaesthesia should in some cases be discussed with the surgeon. Many operations may be performed under some form of local anaesthesia, preferably without using adrenaline. Mild sedation remains imperative, as do the aforementioned monitoring procedures. Giving the patient a high flow of pure oxygen to breathe is often beneficial. Vital regulatory mechanisms are the least disturbed with this management. Yet the continuous presence of a competent anaesthetist remains mandatory, in case acute calamities arise.

3. a. Succinylcholine chloride may, especially in repeated doses, lead to considerable increase of the stimulus threshold, resulting in a myocardium not responding at all to the electrical stimulus of the pacemaker. Cases are described in which the heart was unresponsive for 20 minutes! Lupprian and Churchill Davidson (1960) found that after repeated doses of succinylcholine a bradycardia occurred in 21% of normal non-paced individuals (41 patients); in 7 of these subjects cardiac arrest occurred for between 3-7 seconds (2). The bradycardia was not related to the magnitude of the first dose, but rather to the magnitude of the successive doses. It would therefore seem wise not to use succinylcholine in repeated doses, but rather alcuronium (Alloferine), pancuronium (Pavulon) or possibly d-tubocurarine. Alloferine and Pavulon have virtually no side effects on the heart. The histamine releasing activity of d-tubocurarine would make one hesitant to use it in these cases. Gallamine would seem totally unsuitable, because of its parasympatholytic effects.

b. One single dose of succinylcholine in order to facilitate fast endotracheal intubation would not seem to be contra-indicated. The decelerating action of this drug on the heart seems to be largely due to the release of potassium from the muscle cells, reflected by a disturbance of the normal extracellular $1:1$ potassium/calcium balance. A temporary increase of the serum K with a factor 2 to 3 has been described. This effect can be minimised by temporarily increasing the serum Ca^{++} by means of Ca-gluconate or Ca-laevulinate intravenously. Moreover, calcium, by virtue of its favorable positive inotropic action on the heart, will result in an increased contractile force of the ventricular myocardium. It is therefore our routine to inject 100-500 mg of Ca-laevulinate intravenously prior to a dose of succinylcholine. It has been proven that hyperpotassemia causes an elevation of the stimulus threshold of the myocardium. Surawicz et al. (1965) found a tenfold increase in the threshold after increasing the serum K from 4.0 to 7.1 mEg/l in a pacemaker patient (3).

Especially in intermittent pacemaker failure it is essential to be informed about the serum K/Ca ratio. An elevated threshold may sometimes be lowered by an intravenous Isuprel drip (1-5 mg in 500 ml glucose 5%) or by calcium salts. It can also be superceded by increasing the voltage of the pacemaker impulse, but this is not possible with all pacemakers. An elevated serum K may be lowered by giving glucose and insulin by intravenous drip.

4. During anaesthesia ventricular extra-systoles may occur. These are proof of increased irritability of the myocardium especially if they are multifocal.
   The following causative factors should be considered:

a. hypoxia of the myocardium
b. hypercapnia
c. disturbance of K/Ca balance
d. disturbance of autonomic nervous system balance toward the sympathetic side.

Hypoxia and/or hypercapnia will lead to an increase of circulating cathecholamines; this lowers the stimulus threshold with increased chance of ventricular extra systoles, ventricular tachycardia and even ventricular fibrillation. This holds true for any anaesthesia in general. In a pacemaker patient these aberrant cardiac actions may indicate that a change in threshold has occurred by way of one of the just mentioned mechanisms. In order to avoid hypoxia and/or hypercapnia it is essential to intubate these patients and ventilate them optimally under capnographic control with a gas mixture containing at least 30% oxygen. It would seem wise to avoid anaesthetic gases, vapours or drugs that influence the autonomic nervous system balance or K/Ca ratios to any important degree; therefore trichloroethylene (tachycardia), ether (adrenergic effect), chloroform, cyclopropane (arrhythmias) and high concentrations of halothane (Penthrane) (arrhythmias, hypotension) would all seem contra-indicated.

In case of arrhythmias occurring during halothane anaesthesia, the halothane concentration should be lowered or turned off: in case arrhythmias still persist lignocaine 50 mg i.v., procaine amide 100-500 mg or practolole (Eraldine) up to 5 mg i.v. should be given after excluding other possible causative factors (hypoxia, etc.).

5. *Cardiac output = stroke volume × heart rate*
In order to keep his cardiac output normal the patient can only make use of his cardiac stroke volume. The output of the left heart depends on the venous return to the right heart; if that is decreased (an increase in parasym-

pathetic tone, peripheral vasodilatation, loss of circulating blood volume) a lowered cardiac output will result, with all its consequences for the various organ systems; most important in this respect are cerebral, coronary, hepatic and kidney circulation. The anaesthetist should therefore prevent the decrease of venous return to the right heart, or act immediately in case it does occur. One should consider the use of parasympatholytics, negative phase in positive pressure ventilation, elevation of the legs or the Trendelenburg position. Blood loss should be replaced at once. As a good monitor of this the central venous pressure should be measured continuously. Because of the danger of a high potassium level in old donor blood, the use of fresh blood is preferred.

C. SUGGESTED ANAESTHETIC MANAGEMENT

1.
a. Thorough knowledge of
   i   the patient's vital systems, acid-base balance and electrolytes and
   ii the type of pacemaker and pacemaker's performance.
b. *Premedication*:
   i   Diazepam (Valium) 0.1 mg/kg i.m. 1 hour pre-operatively
       or
       Promethazine (Phenergan) 0.5 mg/kg i.m. 1 hour pre-operatively.
   ii Atropine 0.5 mg s.c. 30 mins. pre-operatively.
       In patients over 70 years of age this may be reduced to about 0.005 mg/kg s.c.

The premedications should preferably be given in a pre-anaesthetic ward, where the patient (already under monitoring) is under constant supervision of an anaesthetist.

c. Pre-oxygenation by face mask for 5-10 minutes with a high flow of oxygen (10-15 1/min.) without rebreathing.
d. Monitoring of E.C.G. and plethysmogram.
e. Wide bore intravenous canula.
f. If tolerated by the patient: central venous pressure should be set up.
g. Multiple, repeated, blood pressure readings as zero-reference for pre-operative measurement.

2. Induction and maintenance of anaesthesia
a. Not more than a sleep dose of a short acting barbiturate such as thiopentone (Penthotal) should be used. One should remember that the circulation in

these patients may be slower than normal, so that an overdose is easily given with all it's possible side effects. *Patience* is of utmost importance: we should not hurry the patient to his grave!

b. It is in all cases mandatory that the patient be ventilated artificially in order to ensure optimal gaseous exchange. Therefore the patient should be intubated and relaxed with muscle relaxants. This will allow us to keep the anaesthesia more superficial and thus to keep the patient's own regulatory mechanisms as undisturbed as possible. As stated before a single dose of succinylcholine would probably not harm the patient, but, in view of the resultant disturbance in the K/Ca balance, it is preferable to use:

i. Pancuronium-bromide (Pavulon) in a dosage of 0.05-0.07 mg/kg i.v.
    or
ii. Diallyl-bis-nortoxiferin (Alloferin) in a dosage of 0.15 mg/kg i.v. followed about two minutes later by endotracheal intubation.

c. The anaesthetic gas mixture should contain at least 30% oxygen in nitrous oxide. If necessary one could add 1/8-1/4% of halothane to this mixture, but often this is not needed. Nitrous oxide 70% will result in anaesthesia, amnesia and moderate analgesia. It will not disturb autonomic nervous system balance, nor influence the distribution of the circulating blood volume. The required total pulmonary ventilatory minute volume should be calculated for each patient. Ventilation should be monitored with and regulated on the basis of a continuous capnogram.

d. The moderate analgesia of 70% nitrous oxide might necessitate the use of additional analgesics.

We prefer small fractionated doses of nico-morphine (Vilan) 0.05-0.10 mg/kg i.v. This drug has virtually no effect on circulation and blood pressure regulation; it has no effect on smooth muscle sphincters or on the motility of the bowel. These factors seem important especially in older people. It furthermore has no respiratory depressant effect post-operatively when given in the mentioned dosage. No interaction with other drugs is known.

e. One should be very careful in changing the patient from the supine position. As is the case in patients under anaesthesia for mitral commissurotomy or pericardiectomy, these pacemaker patients have a fixed cardiac output and one has to balance on a tightrope.

Shifts in position, especially lateral decubitus or jack knife positions may be accompanied by a tremendous fall in blood pressure, resulting from a diminished venous return. These shifts should be made extremely gradually, and in case hypotension occurs, the patient should be turned on his back again.

Short acting plasma volume expanders should then be given, after which (with the central venous pressure as a guide) a shift of position may be tried again.

Abnormal positions may also cause a break in an electrode or the electrode might be pulled out of the battery by traction. The surgeon should have exact knowledge of the place of the electrodes; they might be damaged by his instruments (knife, retractors, etc.). If the patient is to be operated in a position other than the supine position it would seem wise to test the behaviour of the pacemaker and the circulation in that position on the day before surgery.

f. Any loss of blood during the operation should immediately be restored. It may often appear necessary to 'over-transfuse' the patient, preferably with a short acting volume expander (e.g. low molecular dextran).

g. At the end of anaesthesia the action of muscle relaxants should always be reversed.

h. A special problem is the use of electrocautery in patients with cardiac pacemakers.

Electrocautery may trigger ventricular fibrillation or, in case of 'demand' pacemakers, result in failure to give off impulses. Most fixed rate pacemakers are less sensitive in this respect than are 'demand' and 'atrial triggered' pacemakers.

Bipolar pacemakers are less dangerous than the unipolar ones. If electrocautery is necessary the ground plate should be as far remote as possible from the pacemaker.

Also the total grounding of all electronic monitoring equipment should be such, that the development of electrical circuits within the patient (with possible pacemaker interference) is impossible.

During the use of electrocautery the electrocardioscope is either switched off or not interpretable, therefore it is essential to use a simple plethysmoscope (e.g. Cotel-Keating) during that time.

i. Acute severe hypotension, not resulting from massive blood loss or extreme vagotonia, should, in these patients be treated as a cardiac arrest. Ventilation with 100% oxygen and external cardiac massage are immediately indicated.

In case of asystole we are dealing with a pacemaker failure; the myocardium then should be paced by a percutaneously or intravenously introduced electrode.

Needless to say that these instruments should be present in the operating room, in good functioning order (test them first!), prior to induction of anaesthesia.

In the case of ventricular fibrillation external D. C. defibrillation should be performed immediately.

Drugs that should always be at hand, as pointed out earlier, are lignocaine (50 mg i.v.), procainamide (100-500 mg), practolole (Eraldine) (up to 5 mg i.v.), Isuprel, and vasopressors such as adrenaline and mephentermine.

D. REQUIREMENTS

In general the following requirements should be met during anaesthesia for patients with cardiac pacemakers:

1. Optimal precautions and complete knowledge of vital systems and pacemaker performance.
2. Optimal monitoring of vital systems.
3. Keep cardiac output (venous return) normal.
4. Ensure that the patient is normovolemic.
5. Guarantee proper gaseous exchange (capnograph).
6. Keep autonomic nervous system in balance.
7. Keep K/Ca ratio in balance.
8. Respect the pacemaker and electrodes, and ensure that others do so.
9. Avoid sudden shifts in body position.
10. Try to avoid the use of electrocautery.

REFERENCES

1. Various authors on clinical aspects of long-term cardiac pacing. *Annales de Cardiologie et d'Angéiologie* 20, 4, 285 (1971).
2. Lupprian, K. A. & Churchill Davidson, H. C., Effect of suxamethonium on cardiac rhythm. *Brit. Med. J.* 11, 1774 (1960).
3. Surawicz, B., Chlebos, H., Reeves, J. T. & Gettels, L. S., Increase of ventricular excitability threshold by hyperpotassemia: possible cause of internal pacemaker failure. *J. Amer. med. Ass.* 191, 1049 (1965).

PART TWO

MUSCLE RELAXANTS

NEW CONCEPTS OF THE ACTION OF MUSCLE RELAXANTS

S. A. FELDMAN

INTRODUCTION

Just over 225 years ago, de la Condamine (1) set out on a voyage of exploration to Equador. When he returned from his journey he brought back to Leiden a specimen of the South American arrow poison, curare. Subsequently, the Abbé Fontana (1785) used this specimen to perform the earliest recorded pharmacological experiments with this drug. He demonstrated it was harmless if taken orally or inhaled, but poisonous if injected through broken skin. This was the very beginning of research into the pharmacodynamics of the muscle relaxants. This is the story which I intend to pursue in this presentation in an effort to relate pharmacology to clinical experience in the hope that there will emerge a rational basis for our use of these drugs.

Claude Bernard (2) established that the muscle relaxants acted to block nervous impulses from reaching the muscle and effecting muscle contraction. Following the demonstration by Dale (3) and Dale and Feldberg (4) that acetylcholine was responsible for this transmission and that its effects were blocked by curare, it was proposed that curare acted by occupying the cholinergic receptor site, like a key in a lock. The quarternary ammonium groups of the curare were envisaged as locking into a receptor site on the post junctional membrane of the neuromuscular junction.

This theory was challenged by Paton and Zaimis (5) who proposed a dynamic theory of competition in which they postulated 'competitive antagonists' such as curare competing with acetylcholine for available receptor sites. This dynamic state can be represented as

$$y = \frac{(c)}{1 + (c) + (a\ ch)} \qquad y = \text{degree of receptor occupancy.}$$

For this theory to be accepted one must be able to demonstrate:

1. that the degree of receptor occupancy parallels the concentration of curare. $y \propto (c)$,

2. that if the ratio of curare to acetylcholine is kept constant there is a constant degree of receptor occupancy. $y \propto \dfrac{(c)}{(a\ ch)}$

In 1961 Paton (6) modified this concept by introducing the 'Rate Theory'. This proposed that drug activity is associated with its association with a receptor site and that its rate of association may differ from its rate of disassociation. By this means it is possible for a drug to temporarily occupy a receptor site thus prolonging its action and causing it to prevent the access of acetylcholine. This represents 'affinity'.

$$\text{Thus } C + R \; \underset{K_2}{\overset{K_1}{\longrightarrow}} \; CR$$

where K_1/K_2 = affinity constant of C = K_c.

This concept modifies the original competition theory and we now have

$$y = \frac{Kc(c)}{1 + Kc(c) + Ka(a\ ch)} \qquad Ka = \text{affinity constant acetylcholine.}$$

Paton envisaged a dynamic state of association and disassociation, however, if the time constant of assocation differs greatly from that of disassociation, it is necessary to invoke a change of entropy of the system, this might take the form of drug-receptor bonds with specific energy values.

Evidence has been forthcoming to support the competition theory with regard to the action of atropine and acetylcholine on the guinea pig gut (Paton and Rang) (7) and over limited dose range, Jenkinson (8) showed a relationship between ionophoretically applied pulses of carbachol and curare and the degree of paralysis in single muscle fibre units. However, it has become increasingly apparent that in clinical circumstances it is unlikely that effect competition can exist between an agonist like acetylcholine that is destroyed in a fraction of a millisecond and a long acting stable antagonist like curare, Dermot Taylor (9), Ariëns et al. (10).

Although the kinetics of action of drugs at the beta adrenergic receptors of the heart (11) and the muscarinic receptors have been studied (12), it has also become increasingly evident that at the myoneural junction physical barriers, such as the perineural sheath, impose diffusion barriers in the biophase, with time constants that are of such a magnitude, that it is not possible to determine the rates of association and disassociation. Even if it

were possible, the results would not be directly applicable to the clinical situation. Waud (13) suggests that it is probable that the difficulties in access of curare, dimethylcurare and gallamine are the limiting factors in the onset of their action and hence true affinity constants are impossible to determine. In clinical practice the concentration gradient of the drug, the H^+ concentration, local ionic constituents, blood flow and capillary permiability would all affect this overall biophase time and the access to the receptor site.

To obtain meaningful values for the affinity of the muscle relaxants in the clinical circumstances in which they are used, we have studied this problem in man, utilising a technique which allowed us suddenly to lower the blood level whilst observing the degree of paralysis produced by the muscle relaxant. Although the rate of association could not be accurately ascertained by this technique, the rate of recovery of neuromuscular function could be studied quantitatively.

METHOD (14)
Physically fit patients undergoing elective surgery co-operated in this investigation. They were anaesthetised using minimal thiopentone, nitrous oxide and oxygen and 0.5% halothane. A force transducer mounted in a bicycle handle was used to measure the force of contraction of the adductor pollucis longus muscle (15) (Fig. 1). The ulnar nerve was stimulated using subcutaneous needle electrodes with either a Burroughs Wellcome stimulator or a Palmer nerve stimulator. A blood pressure cuff was placed around the upper arm of the patient and an indwelling needle was inserted into a vein on the dorsal surface of the hand. The nerve was stimulated at frequency 0.2Hz. and when a steady response was obtained the cuff was inflated to 200 mm Hg. Twenty millilitres of saline containing either 3 mg curare or 8 mg gallamine, was injected rapidly into the indwelling needle. This was followed by a rapid onset of paralysis as the fluid distended the veins and spread in a retrogade fashion into the tissues. After three minutes the cuff was deflated, causing the blood level of drug in the arm under study to fall from its previous high level to near zero as continuity with the systemic circulation was re-established.

Control experiments established that three minutes of inflation of the cuff did not effect neuromuscular conduction or sensitivity to the relaxant drugs.

RESULTS

Fig. 2 illustrates a typical result using 3 mg curare. There is a rapid onset of curarisation (25 to 75% effect achieved in 0.8 min.). This is followed by a very slow recovery phase *in spite of the fall of blood curare concentration to virtually zero*. In six experiments the mean time for 25 to 75% recovery was 15.6 min. S.D. ± 2.01.

In a further investigation on two of those patients to whom a dose of 20 mg and 30 mg of curare was subsequently administered, the time for 25 to 75% recovery was 17 min. and 22 min. (Table 1). This indicated that the rapid diminution of blood curare only marginally affected the recovery time

Table 1. 25% to 75% recovery times at 'low' and 'high' ECF concentrations.

	Isolated arm 'low' ECF conc.	Whole body 'high' ECF conc.
D-tubocurare	15.6 ± 2.01	17 min. - 20 mg
		22 min. - 30 mg
Gallamine	9.6 ± 0.55 min.	10.5 min. - 100 mg
		12.0 min. - 160 mg

once curarisation had been obtained and that once curare has associated with the receptor its disassociation is not controlled by the blood curare level, provided this is not maintained abnormally high.

Fig. 3 illustrates the results following the injection of 8 mg gallamine. The mean 25 to 75% recovery time of eight experiments was 9.6 min. SD ± 0.55 min. This compared with 10.5 min. in one patient who subsequently received 100 mg gallamine and 12.0 min. in a patient to whom 160 mg of gallamine was administered (Table 1). As with curare, lowering the blood gallamine acutely did not produce a rapid reversal of neuromuscular block, which persisted for almost as long as the block in patients in whom the blood level was not lowered. Thus the receptor occupancy was not proportional to the plasma gallamine level. These experiments indicate that the degree of paralysis produced depends upon the peak plasma level of the drug and that subsequent recovery is independent of the rate of lowering the plasma concentration. This shows a very high affinity constant for curare and gallamine.

These experiments were repeated using decamethonium 0.5 mg in 20 ml of saline. As can be seen in Fig. 4, the 25 to 75% recovery time for this drug was very short. The mean time for the establishment of 25 to 75% paralysis was 0.9 ± S.D. 0.3 min. and that for recovery was 2.56 + 0.28. This recovery

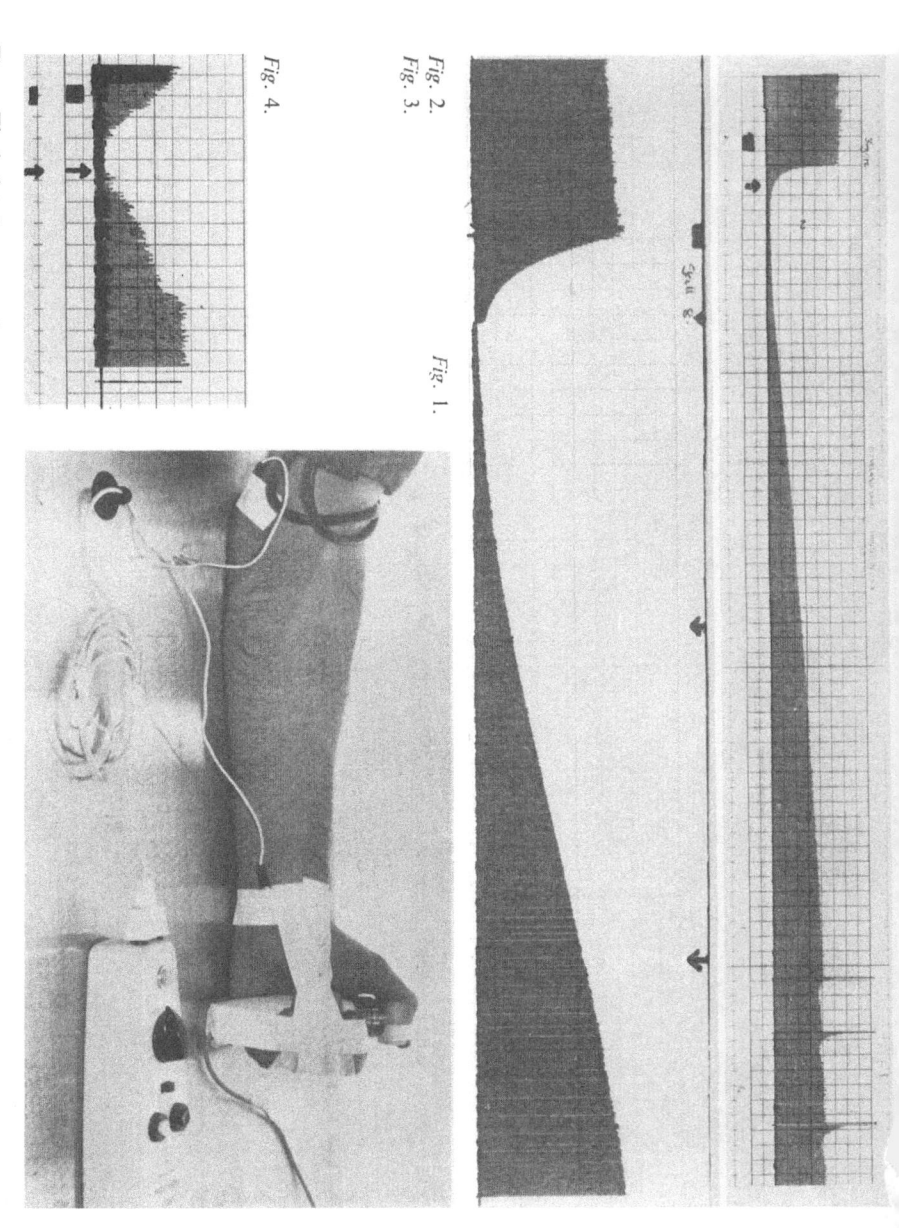

Fig. 1.   The isolated arm experiment.

Fig. 2.   Recovery slope following injection 3 mg d-tubocararine into isolated arm;   ■ injection started;   → cuff released
each sq = 1 min.

Fig. 3.   Gallamine, recovery slope following injection of 8 mg gallamine into isolated arm;   ■ injection started;
→ cuff released; each sq = 1 min.

Fig. 4.   C10 0.5 mg in isolated arm: ■ injection;   → released cuff: 1 sq = 1 min.

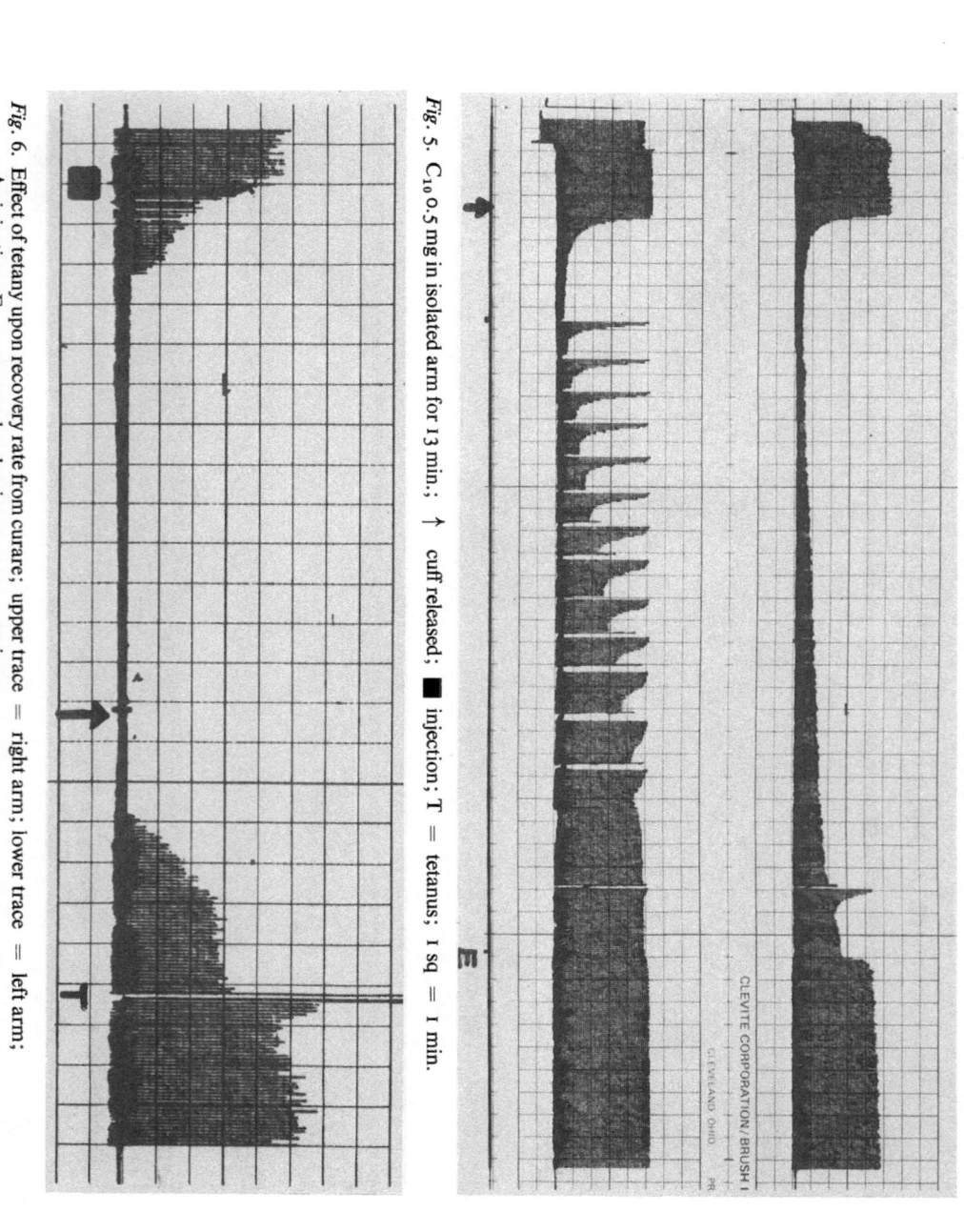

Fig. 5. C_{10} 0·5 mg in isolated arm for 13 min.; → cuff released; ■ injection; T = tetanus; I sq = I min.

Fig. 6. Effect of tetany upon recovery rate from curare; upper trace = right arm; lower trace = left arm; → injection; E = 10 mg edrophonium; I sq = I min.

time is commensurate with the physical washout time from the biophase. It would appear that recovery of neuromuscular conduction following paralysis with a depolarising drug such as decamethonium *is dependent on its plasma concentration* and that it therefore has a low affinity constant.

The experiment with decamethonium was repeated with the cuff inflated for 13 min. instead of 3 min. This produced a different pattern of recovery (Fig. 5). We now have an initial rapid recovery phase followed by a stage of slow recovery. During this slow recovery phase post-tetanic potentiation can be demonstrated. By maintaining the decamethonium in contact with the receptor for a further 10 min. a significant amount of the drug has become fixed and as a result acts as a curare like antagonist to acetylcholine. This suggests that decamethonium is capable of reacting with the receptor in two ways: One is to form a loose association with a low affinity, and as such is acting like acetylcholine (Phase I), the other is a reaction with a long time constant, to form a strong link with the receptor and so to become curare like (Phase II).

REVERSAL OF CURARISATION

Having established that rapidly lowering the blood level does not itself reverse the action of curare, it is necessary to consider the role of acetylcholine in this process. Experiments were performed upon lightly anaesthetised patients to whom no relaxant had been administered. A force transducer was placed in both hands and both ulnar nerves stimulated. A small dose of curare was administered into the jugular vein causing both arms to become paralysed. When recovery had started, one arm was subjected to bursts of tetanic stimuli at $30H_2$ every minute in addition to Faradic stimulation. It can be seen from Fig. 6 that the arm that received the bursts of tetany, and with them bursts of acetylcholine release, recovered far quicker. As acetylcholine is hydrolysed in well under 1 millisec, at any point beyond the last burst of tetany, the amount of acetylcholine and curare in both arms must be similar yet the degree of paralysis is different

$$\text{or y is not proportional to } \frac{(c)}{(a.\ ch)}.$$

It appears that acetylcholine can actively displace curare from its bond with the receptor and providing the blood level of curare is sufficiently low, it will not re-associate but pass out from the end plate along a concentration gradient.

DISCUSSION

The theory suggested is that the amount of paralysis produced by a muscle relaxant depends upon the peak plasma level and that recovery from non-depolarising drugs depends upon the rate and hence the quantity of acetylcholine released. It is tempting to suggest that the random release of packets of acetylcholine cause the normal reversal at the end plate. This work suggests that the activity of these drugs can be affected (a) by factors that affect the peak plasma level (magnitude of block) and (b) factors that alter the rate of release of acetylcholine (duration of block).

The depolarising muscle relaxants act like acetylcholine and will therefore be additive with each other and acetylcholine when acting as Phase I blockers. The observation that the development of a Phase II block has a long time constant is in keeping with the results obtained with succinylcholine upon the rabbit heart (16).

Explanations for the observation that non-depolarising muscle relaxants have a high affinity constant in the clinical situation may lie in the primary reaction between chemical groupings, other than the quarternary ammonium, on these steriochemically rigid molecules and the membrane of the post synaptic junction, to produce energy bonding. This property would be present to only a small degree in the less rigid depolarising drugs, hence the initial reaction of these drugs would be between their quarternary ammonium group and the specific 'onium' receptor of the post synaptic membrane. Only after prolonged exposure, or in the presence of an unusual protein configuration of the post synaptic membrane, would these agents form an energy bond and so act like curare.

An alternative explanation for our observations may lie in the anatomical construction of the myoneural junction and the necessity of drugs to pass through a perineural membrane to gain access to the synaptic cleft. It is possible that this membrane may act as a barrier to diffusion of non-depolarising drugs away from the myoneural junction and by maintaining a high local concentration appear to affect the affinity constant of these agents. In these circumstances it would be necessary to postulate that acetylcholine assisted the egress of non-depolarising relaxants through this membrane.

SUMMARY

In the intact human non-depolarising muscle relaxants appear to become bound to the receptor site from which they are dispersed by acetylcholine.

Depolarising drugs are agents that act like acetylcholine and do not become bound to the receptor site. Providing they are kept in contact with the receptor they have the ability to become bound, but this reaction has a long time constant, hence a Phase II block will only occur after prolonged exposure to the drug.

REFERENCES

1. De la Condamine, C., *Relation abrégée d'un voyage dans l'interieur de l'Amérique meridionale*. Paris 1745.
2. Bernard, C., *C. R. Soc. Biol. (Paris)* 2, 195 (1851).
3. Dale, H. H., Chemical transmission of nerve impulses. *Brit. Med. J.* 1, 835 (1934).
4. Dale, H. H. & Feldberg, W., Transmission at motor nerve ending in voluntary muscle. *J. Physiol.* 81, 39 (1934).
5. Paton, W. D. M. & Zaimis, E. J., Methonium compounds. *Pharmacol. Rev.* 4, 219 (1952).
6. Paton, W. D. M., A theory of drug action based on the rate of drug-receptor combination. *Proc. roy. Soc. B* 154, 21 (1961).
7. Paton, W. D. M. & Rang, H. P., The uptake of atropine and related drugs by intestinal smooth muscle of guinea pig, in relation to acetyl choline receptors. *Proc. roy. Soc. B* 163, 1 (1965).
8. Jenkinson, D. M., The antagonism between tubocurarine and substances which depolarize the motor end-plate. *J. Physiol.* 152, 309 (1960).
9. Dermot Taylor, B., The mechanism of action of muscle relaxants and their antagonists. *Anesthesiology* 20, 439 (1959).
10. Ariens, E. J., Rossum, J. M. van & Simonis, A. M., A theoretical basis of molecular pharmacology. *Arzneimittel-Forsch.* 6, 282 (1956).
11. Paton, W. D. M., Adrenergic receptors viewed in light of general receptor theories. *Ann. N.Y. Acad. Sci.* (1966).
12. Rang, H. P., The kinetics of action of acetyl choline antagonists in smooth muscle. *Proc. roy. Soc. B* 164, 488 (1966).
13. Waud, D. R., The rate of action of competitive neuromuscular blocking agents. *J. Pharm. exp. Therap.* 158, 99 (1967).
14. Feldman, S. A. & Tyrrell, M. F., A new theory of the termination of action of the muscle relaxants. *Proc. roy. Soc. B* 63, 692 (1970).
15. Tyrrell, M. F., A method of measuring the force of adduction of the thumb. *Anaesthesia* 24, 426 (1969).
16. Goat, V. A. & Feldman, S. A., Action of succinylcholine upon the isolated rabbit heart. in press (1971).

THE ACTION OF MUSCLE RELAXANTS
ON CHOLINERGIC MECHANISMS IN THE HEART

V. A. GOAT

Muscle relaxants have relatively few side effects when they are used in the correct dosage in man, as long as adequate ventilation is maintained. However, actions of these drugs may be produced at sites other than the myoneural junction, and these side effects may be accentuated by many factors including the concentration of the drug used, and also the clinical status of the patient.

There have been many reports of changes in heart rate following the use of muscle relaxants in man, both with depolarising and non-depolarising drugs (1, 2, 3). It has been shown that in the intact dog d-tubocurarine chloride is able to partially block the cardiac effects of electrical stimulation of the vagus nerve, and Riker and Wescoe (4) have shown that gallamine triethiodide completely antagonizes the cardiac action of the vagus in the cat. Bonta and his co-workers (5) working with the intact cat showed that pancuronium bromide was able to prevent the bradycardia associated with electrical stimulation of the vagal nerve, but not that following the injection of exogenous acetylcholine.

Many theories have been put forward in an attempt to explain this vagolytic action of the non-depolarising muscle relaxants. This has resulted in confusion as to the site of action and the nature of the cardiac effects of these drugs. This may be partly due to the fact that these agents have multifocal actions affecting the sympathetic ganglia, muscle tone and ionic transport, making it difficult to assess the effect on the heart in the intact animal. In order to overcome some of these difficulties, an isolated rabbit heart preparation was chosen for a study of the cardiac action of the muscle relaxants. A modified Langendof preparation was used, the heart of an adult rabbit being perfused through the cut end of the proximal aorta with oxygenated Ringer/Locke solution, at a constant temperature and pH. The spontaneous contractions of the heart were recorded by means of a Walton-Brodie strain gauge transducer and displayed on a Brush Clevite recorder.

In order to study the cholinergic mechanisms in this isolated preparation, firstly the reaction of the heart to a control injection of acetylcholine (1 μg) was determined before perfusing the heart with the non-depolarising muscle relaxant. Pancuronium bromide, gallamine triethiodide and d-tubocurarine chloride were used on different preparations. Low concentrations of the relaxant were used initially; the heart perfused with that concentration for twenty minutes before increasing the concentration of drug, in order to determine the lowest concentration able to effect complete antagonism to the negative chronotropic action of 1 μg acetylcholine. The results are expressed as the percentage change in heart rate following the injection of the control injection of acetylcholine; hence 100% means that no antagonism was demonstrated whereas 0% antagonism was complete.

In the following figures the log concentration of
1. pancuronium bromide
2. gallamine triethiodide
3. d-tubocurarine chloride
are plotted against the percentage change in heart rate, demonstrating that a linear relationship can be drawn between these two variables (Figs. 1-3).

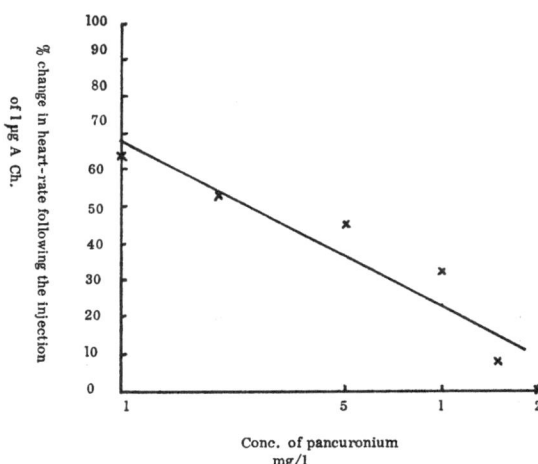

Fig. 1. Antagonism of pancuronium bromide to the negative chronotropic action of 1 μg A. Ch. (Mean values of 7 experiments).

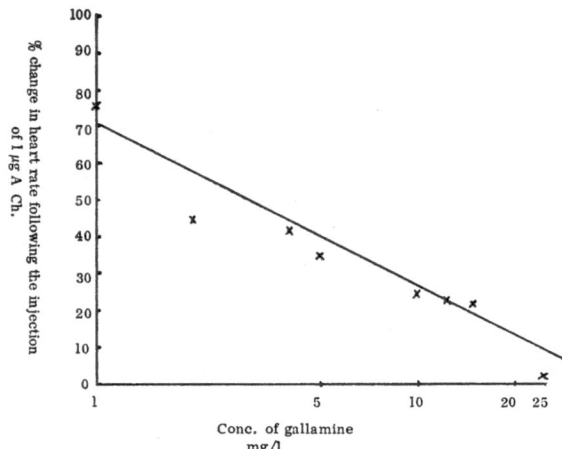

Fig. 2. Antagonism of gallamine triethiode to the negative chronotropic action of 1 μg A. Ch. (Mean values of 8 experiments).

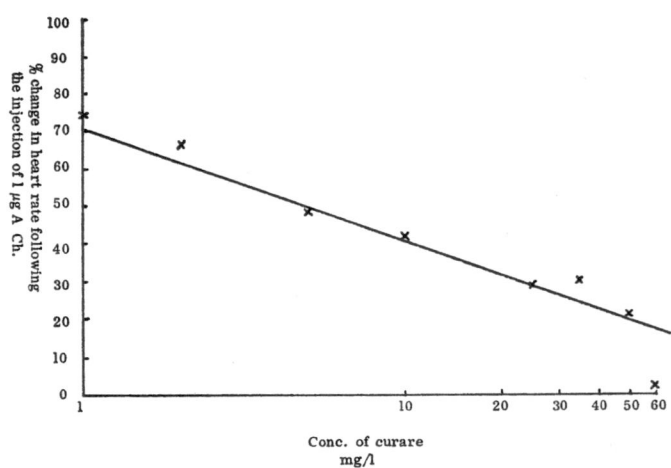

Fig. 3. Antagonism of tubocurarine chloride to the negative chronotropic action of 1 μg A. Ch. (Mean values of 8 experiments).

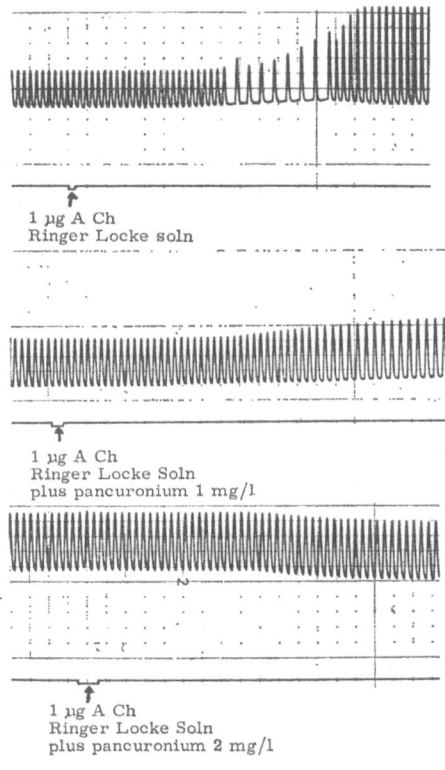

1 µg A Ch
Ringer Locke soln

1 µg A Ch
Ringer Locke Soln
plus pancuronium 1 mg/l

1 µg A Ch
Ringer Locke Soln
plus pancuronium 2 mg/l

Trace 1

Traces 1-3 are typical results from the perfusion of these rabbit hearts.

Trace 1 pancuronium bromide at a concentration of 1 mg/l produced partial antagonism to acetylcholine, and at 2 mg/l the antagonism was complete.

Trace 2 partial antagonism was seen with gallamine triethiodide 12.5 mg/l complete at 25 mg/l.

Trace 3 with d-tubocurarine chloride 50-60 mg/l is required to produce complete antagonism to the negative chronotropic action of 1 µg of acetylcholine.

Pancuronium and gallamine show a cardiac vagolytic action in doses commensurate with peak plasma levels that may be found clinically in man.

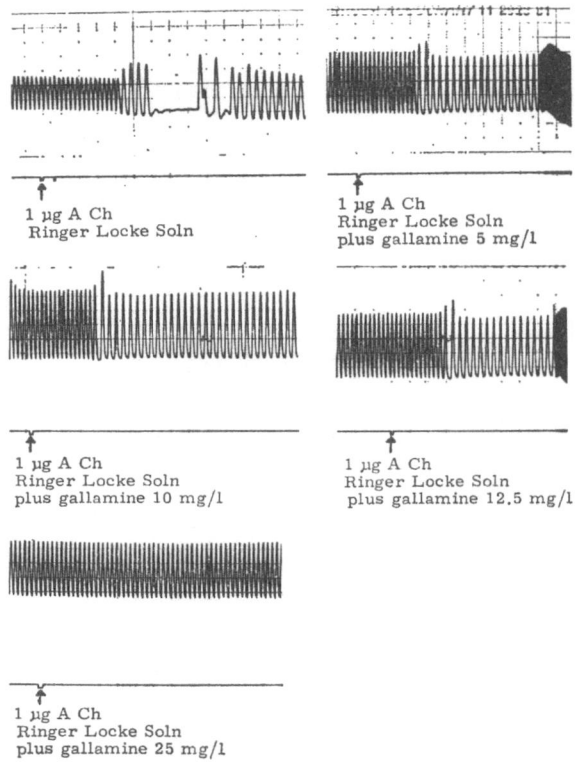

1 µg A Ch
Ringer Locke Soln

1 µg A Ch
Ringer Locke Soln
plus gallamine 5 mg/l

1 µg A Ch
Ringer Locke Soln
plus gallamine 10 mg/l

1 µg A Ch
Ringer Locke Soln
plus gallamine 12.5 mg/l

1 µg A Ch
Ringer Locke Soln
plus gallamine 25 mg/l

Trace 2

However, with d-tubocurarine chloride much higher concentrations were required. If atropine sulphate, a drug known to act at muscarinic cholinergic receptor sites in the atrium, is given prior to the administration of acetylcholine, then no bradycardia is seen (*Trace 4*).

The atropine-like drugs act competitively (6) suggesting direct drug receptor interaction between atropine and the cholinergic receptors. From the preceding results it would appear that pancuronium, gallamine and curare act antagonistically to acetylcholine in a competitive manner. This is strongly suggestive that the non-depolarising muscle relaxants are producing their antagonism to acetylcholine by acting in a similar manner and at the same receptor site as atropine sulphate, at cholinergic receptors in the atrium possibly at the sino-atrial node.

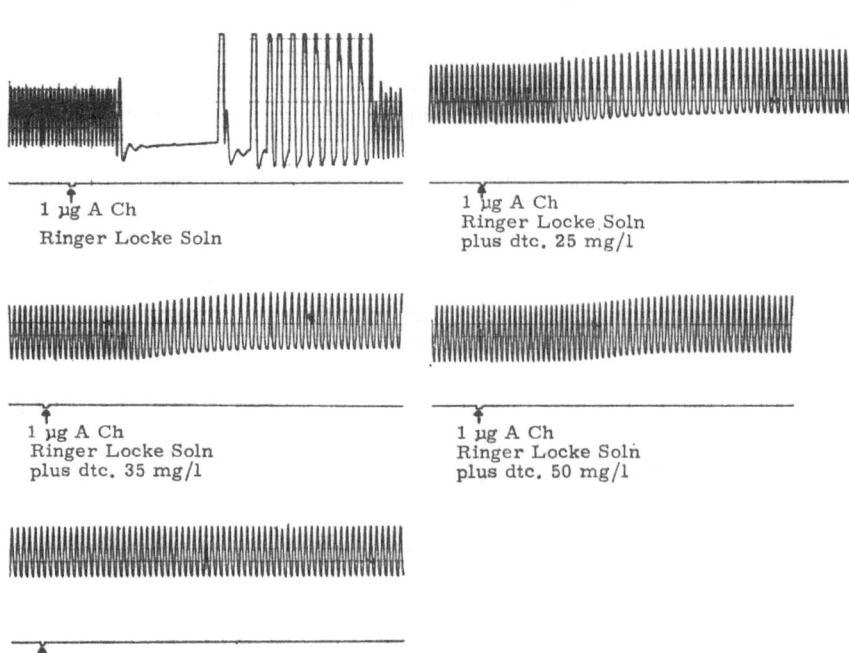

1 µg A Ch
Ringer Locke Soln

1 µg A Ch
Ringer Locke Soln
plus dtc. 25 mg/l

1 µg A Ch
Ringer Locke Soln
plus dtc. 35 mg/l

1 µg A Ch
Ringer Locke Soln
plus dtc. 50 mg/l

1 µg A Ch
Ringer Locke soln
plus dtc. 60 mg/l

Trace 3

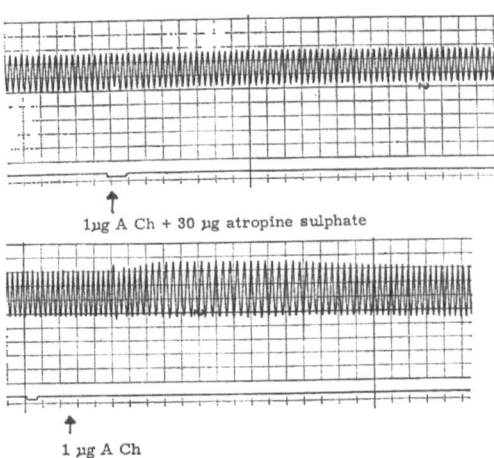

1µg A Ch + 30 µg atropine sulphate

1 µg A Ch

Trace 4

With gallamine triethiodide we have shown that this antagonism persisted for between twenty to fifty minutes after perfusion with the drug has ceased. This is in keeping with Feldman's concept of a high affinity constant or binding for non-depolarising muscle relaxants.

It is well established that acetylcholine produces a biphasic response in the isolated heart. With low concentrations of the drug a negative inotropic and chronotropic response is seen. This direct action of acetylcholine is the one most frequently seen and produced in the preceding experiments. At higher concentrations a positive inotropy and chronotropy may result. This is most readily seen in vagotomized animals (7, 8). The mechanism of this indirect action remains obscure, and it has been suggested that there is release of endogenous catecholamines from intrinsic sympathetic ganglia in the heart (9). However, Appel and Vincenzi (10) working with the isolated sino-atrial node of the rabbit have been unable to confirm the presence of a cholinergic link in the release of catecholamines from this site.

Succinylcholine, a depolarising muscle relaxant commonly used in clinical anaesthesia has a chemical structure resembling two molecules of acetylcholine.

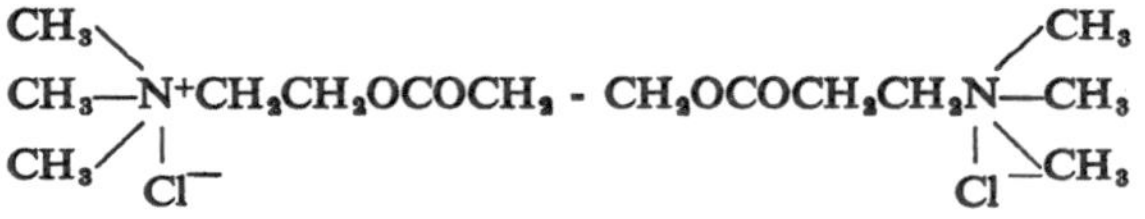

$$CH_3-N^+CH_2CH_2OCOCH_2 - CH_2OCOCH_2CH_2N-CH_3$$

Succinylcholine

$$CH_3-N^+CH_2CH_2OCOCH_3$$

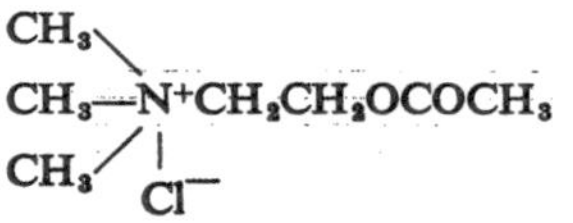

Acetylcholine

Fig. 4.

Numerous cardiac effects both inotropic and chronotropic, have been attributed to the use of this drug. They include bradycardia (11, 12), tachycardia (13, 14, 15), hypotension (16) and hypertension (17). More serious cardiac effects have also been reported, including ventricular arrythmias (18, 19) and ventricular fibrillation and arrest (20, 21).

So from the literature, there appears to be much confusion as to the nature of the cardiovascular effects of succinylcholine, and as might be expected even more confusion as to the mechanism of action of these side effects. The many theories attempting to explain these effects include release of potassium (22), toxic degradation products of succinylcholine (23), and reflex action secondary to stimulation of pressor receptors in the carotid sinus (3).

Clinically, certain groups of patients appear to be more at risk from the cardiovascular side effects of succinylcholine; these include the badly burned subject, small children, digitalized patients and following recent damage to the spinal cord.

In the isolated heart succinylcholine produces a biphasic effect on rate. This is similar to that reported with acetylcholine, low concentrations of the drug (2.5-7.5 mg) producing a bradycardia in the rabbit heart (*Trace 5*), whereas larger amounts of the drug (25-100 mg) resulted in a tachycardia (*Trace 6*).

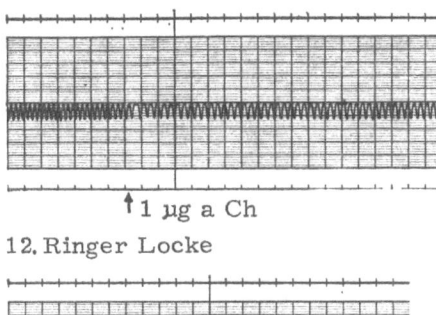

↑ 1 µg a Ch

12. Ringer Locke

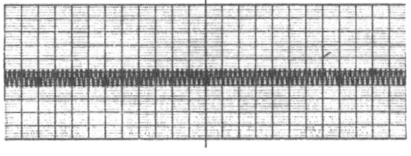

↑ 2.5 mg succinylcholine

13. Ringer Locke

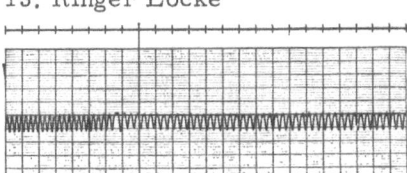

↑ 5 mg succinylcholine

14. Ringer Locke

Trace 5

Trace 5 The effects of low concentrations of succinylcholine on the isolated heart.

Trace 6 The effects of higher concentrations of succinylcholine on the isolated rabbit heart.

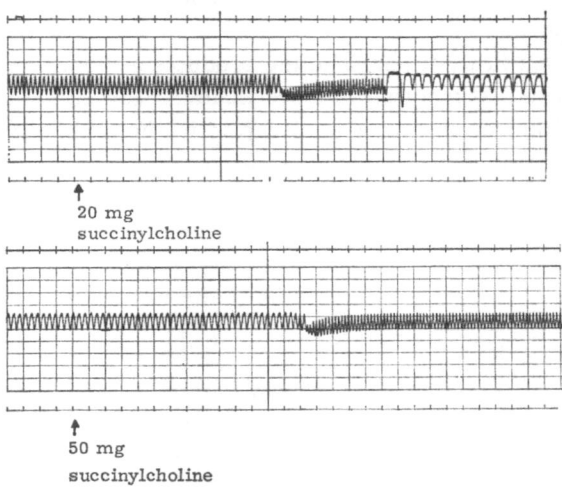

20 mg
succinylcholine

50 mg
succinylcholine

Trace 6

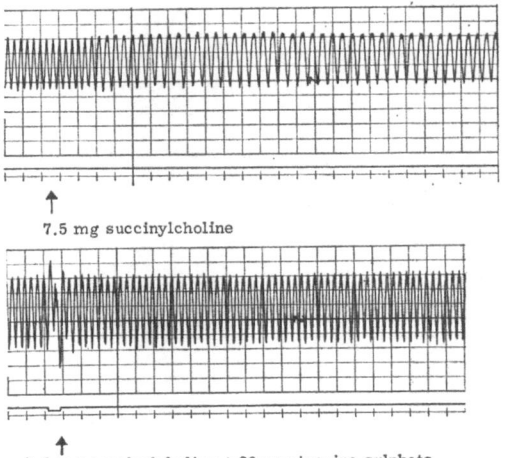

7.5 mg succinylcholine

7.5 mg succinylcholine + 30 µg atropine sulphate

Trace 7

This similarity to acetylcholine is really to be expected if we consider the structural similarity of the two drugs (Fig. 4). The negative chronotropic action of succinylcholine like that of acetylcholine, is also antagonized by atropine sulphate (*Trace 7*), suggesting a similar site of action of the two drugs.

Similarly, if the first group of experiments are repeated using succinylcholine as the cholinergic agonist then complete antagonism to the negative chronotropy produced can be effected by perfusing with pancuronium bromide 2 mg/l (*Trace 8*) or gallamine triethiodide 25 mg/l (*Trace 9*).

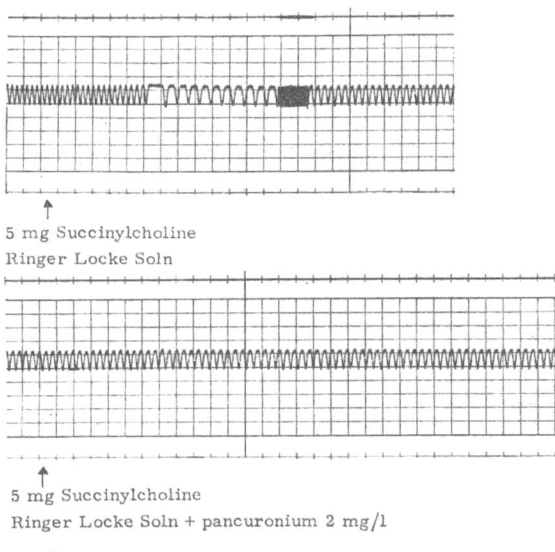

5 mg Succinylcholine
Ringer Locke Soln

5 mg Succinylcholine
Ringer Locke Soln + pancuronium 2 mg/l

Trace 8

This supports the view that succinylcholine is producing its negative chronotropic effect in the same manner as acetylcholine by acting at cholinergic receptors in the isolated heart, possibly at the sino-atrial node.

The conflicting reports as to the nature of the succinylcholine effects on the cardiovascular system in man may partly be explained by this biphasic action of the drug on the isolated heart. It must be remembered that these experiments were done on the isolated rabbit heart, so possible species differences must be considered in attempting to relate these results directly to man.

At the myoneural junction succinylcholine has a dual action. Initially it produces depolarisation acting as a cholinergic agonist, but if the administration of succinylcholine is continued then a non-depolarising type of blockade results. This Phase II block may occur after as little as 2.2-3 mg/kg of drug (24), and the change in the nature of the block has been attributed to the development of receptor bonding, a process that has a long time constant

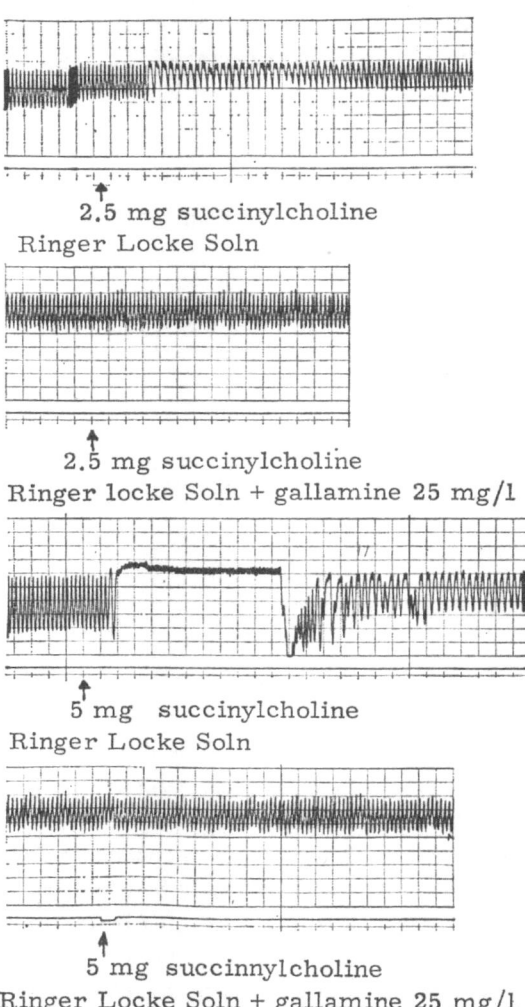

2.5 mg succinylcholine
Ringer Locke Soln

2.5 mg succinylcholine
Ringer locke Soln + gallamine 25 mg/l

5 mg succinylcholine
Ringer Locke Soln

5 mg succinnylcholine
Ringer Locke Soln + gallamine 25 mg/l

Trace 9

with this drug, and therefore is only revealed after exposing the endplate to the drug for prolonged periods (25).

Could this dual block be demonstrated to occur at other cholinergic receptors, for instance those found in the heart? In a further group of experiments the heart was perfused for varying periods of time with different concentrations of succinylcholine ranging from 100 mg/l to 1.5 g/l. The reaction of the heart to the control injection of acetylcholine was established before the perfusion was started, and then repeated at ten minute intervals throughout the perfusion. (*Trace 10* is typical with the onset of antagonism occurring early on and becoming complete thirty five minutes after the perfusion commenced).

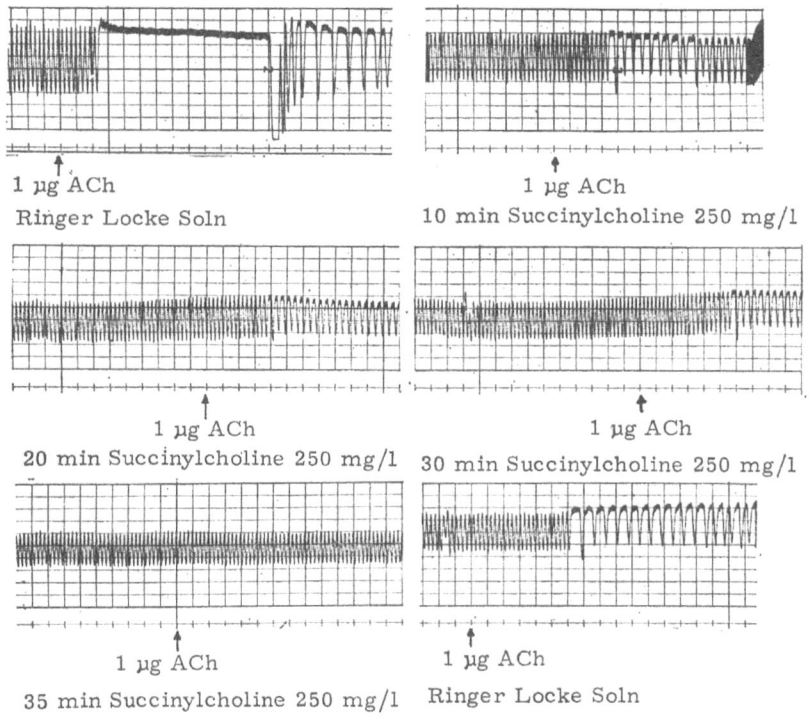

1 µg ACh
Ringer Locke Soln

1 µg ACh
10 min Succinylcholine 250 mg/l

1 µg ACh
20 min Succinylcholine 250 mg/l

1 µg ACh
30 min Succinylcholine 250 mg/l

1 µg ACh
35 min Succinylcholine 250 mg/l

1 µg ACh
Ringer Locke Soln

Trace 10

To demonstrate that this antagonism was true and not due to the development of tachyphylaxis of the heart to acetylcholine, the heart was re-perfused
with Ringer/Locke solution for a ten minute period at the end of each experiment and rechallenged with acetylcholine. This produced an effect
similar in degree to that obtained before the perfusion was commenced. The
results are shown graphically in figure 5 with the percentage change in heart
rate plotted logarithmically against time in minutes from the onset of the
succinylcholine perfusion. The mean values of 14 experiments are plotted
and a direct relationship between the duration of perfusion and the antagonism to the negative chronotropic effect of acetylcholine can be shown. In
other words, a dual block is appearing, succinylcholine is acting in a similar
manner to the non-depolarising muscle relaxants in the isolated heart.

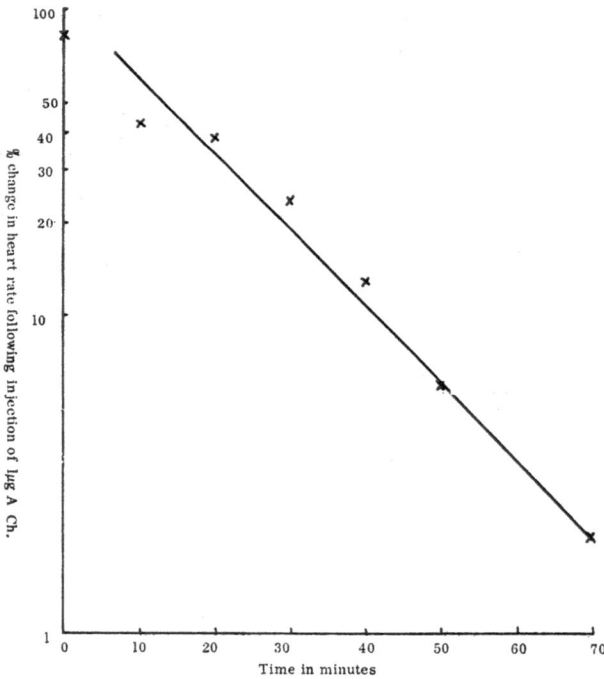

Fig. 5. The relationship between the onset of antagonism to acetylcholine with the duration of perfusion with succinylcholine. (Results are the mean values of 14 experiments).

If, however, the concentration of succinylcholine used in mg/l is plotted against the percentage change in heart rate following the injection of 1 μg acetylcholine, then no relationship between these variables can be demonstrated (Fig. 6).

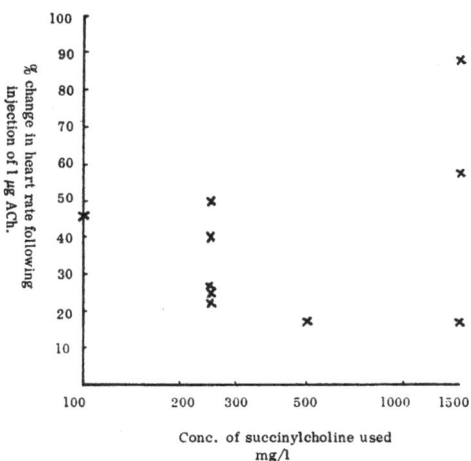

Fig. 6. The relationship between concentration of succinylcholine and the onset of dual block. (Mean values of 14 experiments after perfusion for 20 minutes).

In all these experiments there was no overall change in heart rate following perfusion with the non-depolarising muscle relaxants.

Pancuronium	before perfusion	mean 216 (range 200-240)
	after perfusion	mean 228 (range 200-280)
Gallamine	before perfusion	mean 210 (range 180-240)
	after perfusion	mean 197 (range 140-240)
Curare	before perfusion	mean 220 (range 180-260)
	after perfusion	mean 206 (range 180-240)

With the final group of experiments a negative chronotropic response was seen very rapidly after the succinylcholine perfusion had commenced. As the perfusion continued the heart rate returned to around or just slightly above the pre-perfusion values.

This work carried out on the isolated rabbit heart supports the suggestion that the classical concept of muscarinic and nicotinic cholinergic receptors is becoming more artificial (26). The main difference appears to be a quantitative response to the appropriate agonists and antagonists rather than an absolute specific one. In the heart, the non-depolarising muscle relaxants act antagonistically to acetylcholine, the effect being dose dependant. This strongly suggests that these drugs are acting at cholinergic receptors in the heart – those formerly labelled as muscarinic ones. Succinylcholine has the same effect as acetylcholine in the isolated heart, that is it produces its chronotropic effects by acting as a cholinergic agonist at cholinergic receptors probably in the sino-atrial node. If we attempt to correlate the concentration of drug required in man to effect muscle paralysis, with that required to act as a complete vagolytic agent in the isolated rabbit heart, then gallamine and pancuronium appear to be effective at concentrations used in clinical anaesthesia, curare being least efficient; much higher concentrations being required. The production of dual block with succinylcholine at these cholinergic receptors in the heart is very interesting. It appears to be only time dependant; the concentration of drug used appears to have no effect on its development. This cannot be readily explained using the accepted theories of muscle relaxants.

In respect to their response to various agonists and antagonists the cholinergic receptors in the heart would appear to be intermediate in nature to those found in the gut and those seen at the myoneural junction.

REFERENCES

1. Leigh, M. D., McCoy, D. D., Belton, M. K. & Lewis, G. B., Bradycardia following intravenous administration of succinylcholine to infants and children. *Anesthesiology* 18, 698 (1957).
2. Williams, C. H., Deutsch, S., Linde, H. W., Bullough, J. W. & Dripps, R. D., Effects of intravenously administered succinylcholine on cardiac rate, rhythm and arterial blood pressure in anaesthetised man. *Anesthesiology* 2, 947 (1961).
3. Mathias, J. A., Evans-Prosser, C. O. G. & Churchill-Davidson, H. C., The role of the non-depolarising drugs in the prevention of suxamethonium bradycardia. *Brit. J. Anaesth.* 42, 609 (1970).
4. Riker, W. F. Jr. & Wescoe, W. C., The pharmacology of flaxedil with observations on certain analogues. *Ann. N.Y. Acad. Sci.* 54, 3, 373 (1951).
5. Bonta, I. L., Goorissen, E. M. & Derkx, F. H., Pharmacological interaction between pancuronium bromide and anaesthetics. *European J. Pharmacol.* 4, 83 (1968).
6. Rathbun, F. J. & Hamilton, J. T., Effect of Gallamine on cholinergic receptors. *Canad. Anaesth. Soc. J.* 17, 6, 574 (1970).
7. Koppanyi, K. & MacFarlane, M. D., The cholinergic receptor systems of the atria. *Ann. N.Y. Acad. Sci.* 144, 2, 543 (1967).
8. Dempsey, P. J. & Cooper, T., Ventricular cholinergic receptor systems. Interreaction with adrenergic systems. *J. Pharmacol. exp. Ther.* 167, 282 (1969).

9. Burn, J. & Rand., Sympathetic Post Ganglionic Mechanism. *Nature (London)* 184, 163 (1900).
10. Appel, W. C. & Vincenzi, F. F., Effects of hemicholinium on the release of automatic transmitters in the isolated sino-atrial node. *Brit. J. Pharmacol.* 40, 268. (1970).
11. Johnston, M., Relaxants and the human cardiovascular system. *Anaesthesia* 10, 122 (1955).
12. Galindo, A. & Davis, T., Succinylcholine and cardiac excitability. *Anesthesiology* 23, 32 (1962).
13. Beretervide, K. V., Actions of succinylcholine chloride on the circulation. *Brit. J. Pharmacol.* 10, 265 (1955).
14. Conway, C. M., The cardiovascular actions of suxamethonium in the cat. *Brit. J. Anaesth.* 33, 560 (1961).
15. Adams, A. K. & Hall, L. W., An experimental study of the action of suxamethonium on the circulatory system. *Brit. J. Anaesth.* 34, 445 (1962).
16. Paton, W. D. M., The effects of muscle relaxants other than muscle relaxation. *Anesthesiology* 20, 453 (1959).
17. Goodman, L. S. & Gilman, A., *The pharmacological basis of therapeutics.* 3rd. ed. New York 1965.
18. Lupprian, K. G. & Churchill-Davidson, H. C., Effect of suxamethonium on cardiac rhythm. *Brit. Med. J.* 2, 1774 (1960).
19. Vanner, G. K., Loennecken, S. J., Richard, K. E. & Schmucker, H., Repeated cardiac arrest following suxamethonium. In: *Progress in anaesthesiology. Proceedings of the fourth World Congress of Anaesthesiologists, Amsterdam.* p. 770. Amsterdam 1970.
20. Tolmie, J. D., Joyce, T. H. & Mitchell, G. D., Succinylcholine danger in the burned patient. *Anesthesiology* 28, 467 (1967).
21. Belin, R. P. & Karleen, C. I., Cardiac arrest in the burned patient following succinyl-choline administration. *Anesthesiology* 27, 516 (1966).
22. Stone, W. A., Beach, T. P. & Hamelberg, W., Succinylcholine induced hypertalaemia in dogs with transected sciatic nerves or spinal cords. *Anesthesiology* 32, 515 (1970).
23. Gologorsky, V. A. & Umanov, J. M., The mechanism of succinylcholine effect on heart rate and rhythm. In: *Progress in anaesthesiology. Proceedings of the fourth World Congress of Anaesthesiologists, Amsterdam.* p. 1165. Amsterdam 1970.
24. Katz, R. L., Wolfe, C. E. & Papper, E. M., The non-depolarising neuro-muscular blocking action of succinylcholine in man. *Anesthesiology* 34, 784 (1963).
25. Feldman, S. A. & Tyrrell, M., A new theory of the termination of action of muscle relaxants. *Proc. roy. Soc. Med.* 63, July (1970).
26. Chiou, C. Y., Long, J. P., Potrepka, R. & Spratt, J. L., The ability of various nicotinic agents to release acetylcholine from synaptic vescicles. *Arch. int. Pharmacodynamic Ther.* 187, 88 (1970).

CHANGES OF ACID-BASE BALANCE AND MUSCLE RELAXANTS

J. F. CRUL AND E. J. CRUL*

When studying the effect of acid-base changes on muscle relaxants, one must firstly ask whether changes in these parameters alter neuromuscular transmission and secondly the action of muscle relaxants.

Fig. 1a. Possible sites of action of acid-base change in blood

1. Ionisation of curare molecule
2. Protein binding
3. Plasma cholinesterase activity
4. Excretion – redistribution

Fig. 1b. Possible sites of action of acid-base change in motor units

1. Nerve conduction velocity
2. Acetylcholine liberation by changes in Ca^{++}
3. Resting membrane potential (K^+ intra-extracell)
4. Perfusion endplate
5. Ionisation receptor-molecule
6. True cholinesterase activity
7. Contractility of musclefibers
8. Catecholamines secretion

Figures 1a and 1b, summarize the possible sites of action and it is seen that several factors in the blood and at the motor neurone are altered by acid-base changes. The purpose of this work was to study the overall effect of these changes.

Having accepted that acid-base changes may interfere with muscle contraction and relaxation, it is then important to define the types of changes.

* This work was partially supported by a grant from the National Institute for applied research T.N.O.

There can either be an increase in acids (hydrogen ion donors) or a loss of base – both resulting in acidosis. The reverse alkalosis (or baseosis) is caused either by a respiratory imbalance with a change in the level of carbonic acid in the blood, or by a metabolic disorder in which a change in base or fixed non volatile acid takes place.

It was not known whether it made any difference if the pH changes were primarily extra- or intracellular, metabolic or respiratory, on the effect on the motor system. Also a certain degree of compensation of the primary acid-base change almost always occurs in the extracellular compartment of the living organism. This compensation is even greater within the cell (Fig. 2) (1). Therefore pure states almost never exist.

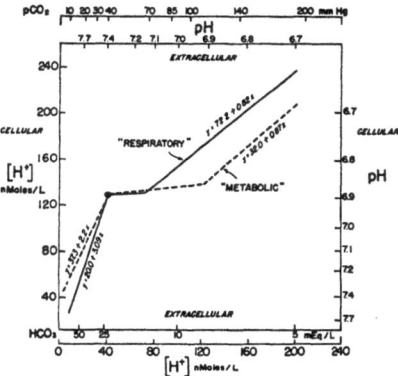

Fig. 2. Intracellular pH changes in relation to extracellular respiratory or metabolic acid-base abnormalities. Note the relative stability of intracellular pH over a certain range of extracellular acidosis, but very little resistance to extracellular alkalosis. With permission taken from Adler, S. et al. (1).

A further complication is the fact that metabolic acid-base disturbances cannot be easily or safely reproduced in man. This makes the study of these effects difficult in the clinical situation of the operating room or the intensive care unit (2). Therefore most researchers resort to animal experiments, and it is from these that most of the data has been collected.

A summary of the results published up to 1969 is given in figure 3. It is apparent that the biggest gaps occur in the study of metabolic acidosis and respiratory alkalosis. The same figure shows that some of the results are contradictory, depending on the technique used and the species selected. Katz (3) has made the greatest contribution about the effect of metabolic

| Agents and authors | Species | Acidosis | | Alkalosis | |
		Respiratory	Metabolic (HCl)	Respiratory	Metabolic
d-tubocurarine					
Kalow	frog		+		—
Gamstorp-Vinnars	rabbit	+	+	—	—
Payne	cat	+	—		+
Utting	dog			—	
Frederickson	cat	+		—	
Katz, Ngai, Papper	cat				—
Johanson-Osgood	cat	+			
Baraka	man	+		—	
Bridenbaugh	man	+		—	
Coleman	man	+		—	
Dundee	man			—	
di-methyl tubocurarine					
Kalow	frog		0		0
Payne	cat	—	—		+
Gamstorp-Vinnars	rabbit	0	0	0	0
Katz, Ngai, Papper	cat				+
Baraka	man			0	+
gallamine					
Osgood-Johansen	cat	—			
Payne	cat	—			+
Katz, Ngai, Papper	cat			+	+
Bridenbaugh	man	—			
succinylcholine					
Johansen-Osgood	cat	0			
Payne	cat	—			
Katz, Ngai, Papper	cat				+
Kronschwitz	man	—		0	+
C 10					
(decamethonium)					
Johansen-Osgood	cat	0			
Payne	cat	—			
Katz, Ngai, Papper	cat				—(0)
alloferine					
Coleman	man				0

Metabolic Alkalosis   by Kalow — NaOH   + = potentiation
             by Gamstorp-Katz — Na_2CO_3 — = antagonism
                  by Payne — $NaHCO_3$ 0 = no effect

Fig. 3. Summary of studies on effects of acid-base changes on muscle relaxants up till 1969.

alkalosis. Since then data has been added by Coleman (4) from human studies and by Hughes (5) from cats.

A long term project was undertaken to fill the gaps in these studies.

TECHNIQUES

Several in vivo and in vitro experiments were carried out in animals and man. They can only be briefly summarized in this report. Cats resemble man most closely in their sensitivity to muscle relaxants, and were used extensively for the animal studies. In order to compare both fast and slow muscles, the anterior tibialis and soleus muscles were studied, as almost pure representatives of these types (Fig. 4). In the latter groups of experiments the respiratory

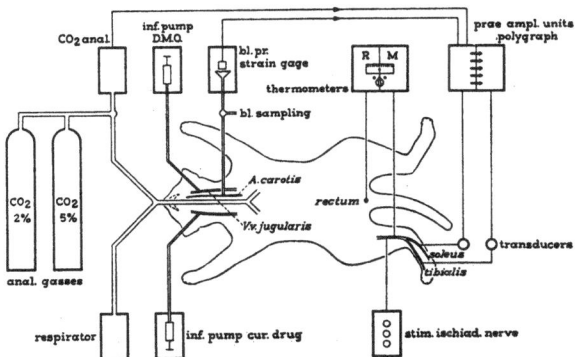

Fig. 4. Experimental set-up for study of effects of acid-base changes on muscle relaxants in cats. Both slow and fast muscle-contractions are studied, with indirect stimulation of the ischiadic nerve. Steady state partial paralysis is instituted by infusion of relaxant drug. Superimposed acidifying or alkalising drugs are infused with another pump. Respiratory changes are caused by hyperventilation or inhalation of 10% CO_2.

muscle of the diaphragm was studied, using a new specially designed technique (Fig. 5). By this method it was possible to study concomitantly the mechanical contractions of three types of muscle in one animal in vivo. Until now this had not been possible.

Also the anterior tibialis muscle of the rat in vivo was studied and the phrenic nerve-diaphragm preparation of the rat (modified Buelbring technique) in vitro, using a double organ bath in order to have a control strip of the same diaphragm.

In man, the mechanical force displacement of the adductor pollicis muscle was observed, using indirect stimulation via the ulnar nerve (Fig. 6). Katz (6) showed that these mechanical contractions were less influenced by

other than curariform drugs, and Botelho (7) found that in partially cur-
arised patients, these contractions most closely reflected the return of
muscle power in the awakening patient. In some experiments the electromyo-

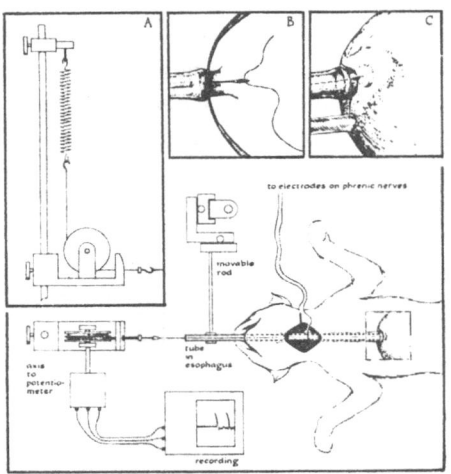

Fig. 5. Technique of studying spontaneous and indirectly evoked contractions of the
diaphragm in the cat. Movements of the diaphragm are transduced by the wire through
the oesophagus to an auxotonic force displacement transducer. Respiration is unimpaired
by this technique and the general condition remains physiological.

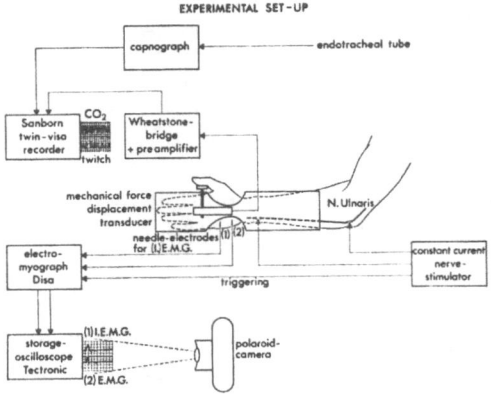

Fig. 6. Set-up of muscle relaxant studies in man. The ulnar nerve is stimulated via subcutaneous needle-electrodes. The contraction of the adductor pollucis muscle is recorded
isometrically. The electromyogram of hypothenar muscles is recorded with a Dysa
electromyograph and recorded on a polaroid camera.

graphic changes in the hypothenar muscles were recorded by means of coaxial needle electrodes.

Since Katz (3) had most recently studied metabolic alkalosis, it was decided to study primarily, the changes caused by respiratory alkalosis and also acidosis, both respiratory and metabolic.

The pitfalls of this type of study are enumerated below. Since many factors can influence the results the possible snags must be carefully studied before choosing a good experimental set-up. A few of the major ones are mentioned here.

1. Careful attention to supramaximal stimulation of the nerve is important. A choice should be made between twitches and tetanic stimulation.

2. Optimal preloading of the muscle tension should be aimed at.

3. A steady state of muscle relaxation should be obtained before the effects of acid-base changes are studied.

4. As far as possible, each animal should be used as its own control, since there is considerable individual variation in the animals' sensitivity to neuromuscular blockade. This can be done by observing the recovery of the contraction height to its original level at the end of the experiment.

5. The choice of drugs used to stimulate the acid-base changes is important, particularly in metabolic studies. An example is the common use of HCl, to produce metabolic acidosis. Not only does it not penetrate across cell membranes, but it also causes brutal circulatory effects, which can influence the end results considerably. It is simpler to produce the respiratory changes; this can be done by hyperventilation or the addition of CO_2 to the inhaled gases. Too high concentrations of CO_2 must be avoided, since this can seriously alter the circulation. Not more than 10% is advocated.

6. In order to study the effects of acid-base changes, the immediate effects must be noted before the compensatory changes have occured.

For this work:

a. Hyperventilation to $PaCO_2$ values of 15-20 mm Hg was used to produce respiratory alkalosis both in animals and man.

b. Inhalation of 10% CO_2 for 10 minutes was used to produce respiratory acidosis in animals.

c. In order to produce metabolic acidosis in animals, DMO was used. This is a weak organic acid, with special features making it the ideal substitute for

normally occurring metabolic acidosis (Fig. 7). Later on, another group
of acids was used, to avoid the direct chemical effect of the drug, in addition to its action as a proton donor. The metabolic acidosis caused by
this drug is summarized in figure 8.

DMO	
5-5-Dimethyl 2,4 oxazolidine dione	
PK	6.13
Ionic strength	0.16
Low toxicity	
No binding to protein	
No entering fat depots	
No metabolism	
Excreted by kidneys	

Fig. 7. DMO a weak organic acid, used to imitate metabolic acidosis, most closely resem-
bles the non-volatile acids produced in the body during this state, but is more stable. It is
widely used in studies on intracellular pH changes.

	pH M $\pm$ S.D.	PCO$_2$ M $\pm$ S.D.	B.E. M $\pm$ S.D.
Before DMO	7.35 $\pm$ 0.06	32.3 $\pm$ 5	— 7.5 $\pm$ 4
After DMO	7.09 $\pm$ 0.08	30.2 $\pm$ 10	—20.6 $\pm$ 4

Fig. 8. Acid-base changes caused by an infusion of DMO in cats.

In all the groups *blank* studies indicate the absence of effect of the *test* dose of
acidifying or alkalinising drug on normal neuromuscular conduction, using
tetanic stimulation. It is not possible to give further details in this short
paper about every separate group of experiments. Where metabolic alkalosis
had not been studied by us, the results of Katz (3) on cats, and Hughes
(which agreed nicely) were added. *Respiratory alkalosis* in *cats* potentiates
the depolarising relaxants and has no effect on the non-depolarisers (Fig. 9).
The new drugs like alcuronium (alloferine) and pancuronium are not influenced by hyperventilation (8, 9). In man *hyperventilation* had little effect on
either group of muscle relaxants, certainly of no major clinical significance
(Fig. 10).

Katz (3) and Hughes (5) agreed that *metabolic alkalosis* had the same effect
on succinylcholine and d-tubocurarine as we found in our studies with respiratory alkalosis. That is succinylcholine was potentiated, d-tubocurarine
weakly antagonized. No work has been done to study the effect of metabolic
alkalosis on the newer muscle relaxants.

Drug	Number	Effects	
		M. tib. ant.	M. soleus
Control	7	None	None
Succinylcholine	13	12 potentiation	5 potentiation
		1 no effect	4 no effect
C 10	7	Potentiation	Potentiation
d-tubocurarine	10	None	None
Alloferine	8	None	None
Total	45		

Fig. 9. Effect of respiratory alkalosis on de-polarising and non-depolarising relaxants in cats.

Drugs	Number	Mean FA_{CO_2} in S.R.	Mean FA_{CO_2} in H.V.	Effect
Controls	6	6.2%	2.4%	50% increase of controls
Succinylcholine	5	6.7%	2.5%	Antagonism
d-tubocurarine	6	5.5%	2.6%	3 no effect
				3 weak antagonism
Alloferine	4	5.5%	2.2%	No effect

Fig. 10. Effect of respiratory alkalosis on depolarising and non-depolarising relaxants in man.

In cats *respiratory acidosis* produced the same effect as *metabolic acidosis* suggesting that as far as neuromuscular blockade is concerned, it does not matter whether the H^+ ions are produced by ventilatory or metabolic disturbances. Depolarising relaxants were strongly antagonized in cats by both types of acidosis (Fig. 11). Of the non-depolarising group, d-tubocurarine was significantly potentiated, but the effect on the newer drugs, pancuronium and alcuronium (alloferine) was negligible.

	Number exp.	Effect
Controls	5	None
Succinyl choline	7	Antagonism
C 10	10	Antagonism
d-tubocurarine	8	1 no reaction
		7 potentiation
Alloferine	8	Weak potentiation
Total	38	

Fig. 11. Effect of metabolic acidosis caused by DMO on depolarising and non-depolarising muscle relaxants.

	Respir. acidosis	Metabol. acidosis	Respir. alkalosis	Metabol. alkalosis
succinylcholine	=	=	++	0
C 10	—	—	+	0
d-tubocurarine	+	++	—	—
Pancuronium	0	0	0	

— = antagonism of block
+ = potentiation of block
0 = no effect

Fig. 12. Effects of metabolic and respiratory acidosis, metabolic and respiratory alkalosis on depolarising and non-depolarising relaxants in cats. A combined summary of our results and those of other authors (Katz, Hughes).

An overall picture of the influence of acid-base balance, on the commonly used relaxants is given in figure 12. Looking at the effects as a whole, only the action of alkalosis and acidosis on the depolarising relaxants and d-tubo-curarine are of clinical importance. As d-tubocurarine becomes replaced more and more by the newer relaxants, which are far less influenced, the role of acid-base changes in clinical anaesthetic practice can be *neglected* for the *non-depolarising* relaxants. The diaphragm behaved identically with the other muscles in these experiments.

In summary – the effect of metabolic or respiratory changes in the acid-base state, on the muscle relaxants, is identical. Depolarising and non-depolarising drugs react in a directly opposite way to acid and alkaline states. For most states and relaxants the effect is minimal.

The *in vitro* preparations produced similar results, even on a quantitative basis, which rules out therise in catecholamine level or circulatory changes as possible causes for the effects. This strongly suggests that with the exception

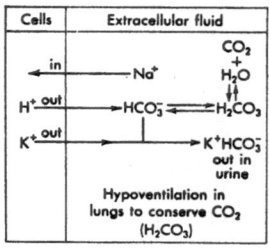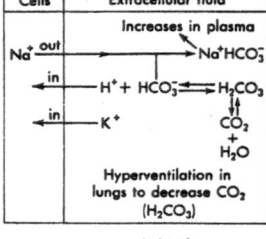

Fig. 13. Shifts of electrolytes during alkalosis and acidosis between the cells and the extracellular fluid. These shifts influence the resting membrane potential directly, and thereby can influence the effect of depolarising and non-depolarising relaxants. With permission taken from: West, E. S. (11).

of d-tubocurarine a common denominator determines these influences, namely the changes in resting membrane potential. According to most theoretical studies, so nicely reviewed in 1963 by Dr. Feldman (10) a co-lecturer of this symposium, it is assumed that after elimination of the other possible factors, these effects are caused by changes in the resting membrane potential.

Changes in both the intra- and extracellular concentration of K^+ are known to follow shifts of H^+ ions into and out of the cell (Fig. 13). As far as we are aware no direct measurements of resting membrane potentials of muscle cells have been made during changes in acid-base balance. This work is being done at present and the results will be reported at a later date.

Finally the importance of the central influences of acid-base changes on muscle activity must be stressed. This is probably one of the major sources of post-operative muscle weakness and should therefore be differentiated from the peripheral effects described here.

REFERENCES

1. Adler, S., Roy, A. & Relman, A. S., Intracellular acid-base regulation. I: The response of muscle cells to changes in CO_2 tension or extracellular bicarbonate concentration. *J. clin. Invest.* 44, 8 (1965).
2. Vourc'h, G., Metabolic acidosis and acute post-operative respiratory insufficiency. In: *Curare. Symposion der Schweizerischen Akademie der Medizinischen Wissenschaften*, 25/26 Juni 1966, Zürich, p. 107. Basel/Stuttgart 1966.
3. Katz, R. L., Ngai, S. H. & Papper, E. M., The effects of alkalosis on the action of neuromuscular blocking agents. *Anesthesiology* 24, 18 (1963).
4. Coleman, A. J., Ripley, S. H., Sliom, C. M. & Knowles, S. L., The influences of carbon dioxide on the neuromuscular blocking properties of tubocurarine chloride and diallyl-nor-toxiferine dichloride (Alloferin Roche) in man. In: *Curare. Symposion der Schweizerischen Akademie der Medizinischen Wissenschaften*, 25/26 Juni 1966, Zürich, p. 98. Basel/Stuttgart 1966.
5. Hughes, R., The influence of changes in acid-base balance on neuromuscular blockade in cats. *Brit. J. Anaesth.* 42, 658 (1970).
6. Katz, R. L., Monitoring of muscle relaxation and neuromuscular transmission. In: Crul, J. F. & Payne, J. P., (eds.) *Patient monitoring*, p. 129. Amsterdam 1970.
7. Botelho, S. Y., Comparison of simultaneously recorded electrical and mechanical activity in myasthenia gravis patients and in partially curarized normal humans. *Amer. J. Med.* 19, 693 (1955).
8. Crul, J. F., In: *Curare. Symposion der Schweizerischen Akademie der Medizinischen Wissenschaften*, 25/26 Juni 1966, Zürich, p. 113. Basel/Stuttgart 1966.
9. Crul, J. F., Studies on new steroid relaxants. In: *Progress in anesthesiology. Proc. 4th World Congress of Anesthesiology.* p. 418. (Int. Congress series, nr. 200), Amsterdam 1970.
10. Feldman, S. A., Effect of changes in electrolytes, hydration and pH upon the reactions to muscle relaxants. *Brit. J. Anaesth.* 35, 546 (1963).
11. West, E. S., *Textbook of biophysical chemistry*. 3rd ed., p. 290. New York 1964.

THE USE OF MUSCLE RELAXANTS IN ANEPHRIC PATIENTS

D. T. POPESCU

Since their introduction into anaesthesia nearly 30 years ago, muscle relaxant drugs have been extensively studied. However, gaps in our knowledge still persist, which explains the appearance of new theories of action still occurring in the literature (1, 2).

The administration of muscle relaxants to patients with healthy kidneys normally presents no problems, although residual curarisation has been reported by Hannington-Kiff (3) after a routine anaesthetic. Most of the published complications following the use of muscle relaxants have occurred in patients with reduced renal function, and this has led to further investigations about their metabolism and elimination.

It is generally accepted that muscle relaxants need to be used cautiously in patients with renal insufficiency. The depolarising agents are reputed to be safe, and Rolly (4) has reported good results with the use of succinylcholine in renal transplantation, whilst some English workers have commented favourably on the use of d-tubocurarine in these cases (5).

Until recently, the use of gallamine has been condemned because this drug is totally removed unmetabolised by the kidneys. However, White (6) has reported the use of this drug, without complications, in patients undergoing bilateral nephrectomies. Other reports appear to disagree with this work (7). Because of this apparent controversy in the literature it was decided to conduct a retrospective study of patients admitted to the University hospital in Leiden for inclusion in the renal transplantation scheme.

All these patients had most or all of the factors in common:

– absence of renal function, or gross renal insufficiency ($\pm$ 100 ml urine/day) necessitating regular haemodialysis.
– severe anaemia.
– instability of water and electrolytic balance.
– repeated anaesthetics during treatment (mean 3.5 range 2-11).

Constant:
- Absence of renal function or gross insufficiency
- Severe anaemia 6.85 gr %   (5-10.8)
- Repeated anaesthesias 3.5   (2-11)
- Lability of water and electrolytes

Often:
- Arterial hypertension
- Recent dialysis – hypovolaemia
              – low serum ch-est
              – low potassium (min. 2.5)
- Before dialysis – hyperhydration
              – acidosis
              – uraemia
              – high potassium (max. 6.8)

Fig. 1. Characteristics of patients.

- hypertension.
- post-dialysis hypovolaemia, low serum cholinesterase and low serum potassium.
- pre-dialysis acidosis, overhydration, uraemia and hyperkalaemia.

These factors would appear to make these patients suitable subjects for assessing the results of muscle relaxants.

EXPERIENCE OBTAINED IN LEIDEN

The first renal transplant to be performed in Leiden took place on 2nd March, 1966. From this time until 15th August, 1971, a total of 106 patients have been included in the transplantation scheme, and 74 kidney transplants performed on 73 patients (1 patient received two transplants). Unfortunately some of the details are missing from the records, but this study is based on the data available.

106 Patients. 417 Anaesthesias

Local anaesthesia	122
General anaesthesia	295
Without relaxant	95
With relaxant	200
Good kidney function	19 times
Relaxants in anephric cases	181

Fig. 2.

The 106 patients underwent 417 anaesthetics, of which 122 were local and
295 general anaesthetics. Muscle relaxants were used on 200 occasions. Of
the remaining 95 general anaesthetics, administered to 50 patients, these included anaesthesia for minor procedures such as the insertion of shunts, and
for procedures not requiring muscle relaxation or where the relaxation was
provided by ether anaesthesia. This included anaesthesia for parathyroidectomy, removal of the transplanted kidney and relaparotomies. 12 Patients
out of the original group had good renal function, and the 19 general anaesthetics administered to these patients for parathyroidectomy, correction
of renal artery, gastrectomies, cholecystectomies and total hip replacement,
were excluded from latter calculations along with the group not receiving
muscle relaxants.

ANAESTHESIA

Premedication varied from intravenous atropine only, to pethidine-atropine,
pethidine-promethazine-atropine, papavaretum-atropine, diazepam-atropine
or thalamonal-atropine.

    The anaesthetics can be put into four groups depending on the main main-
tenance agent used (Fig. 3).

Premedication	Type anaesth.	Maintenance
Atropine	I	Halothane
± Opial		+ N_2O + O_2
± Pethidine	II	Aether +
± Prometha-		Halothane
zine		+ N_2O + O_2
Atropine	III	Methoxyflurane
± Diazepam		+ O_2
Atropine	IV	NLA II
± Thalamonal		

Fig. 3.

Group 1. Halothane, nitrous oxide and oxygen after induction with thiobar-
bitone (kemithal) and succinylcholine.

Group 2. The same as in Group 1, plus the addition of diethyl ether in
order to obtain better analgesia and relaxation. (Groups 1 and 2-174 anaesthetics).

Group 3. Maintained on oxygen-methoxyflurane after induction with propanidid and succinylcholine (100 anaesthetics).

Group 4. Neurolept anaesthesia.

Anaesthesetics administered during the first three and a half years of the survey came into the 1st or 2nd groups, and more recent ones come into group 3 (1½ years) and group 4 (6 months).

When muscle relaxants were used the mean duration of anaesthesia was 152 minutes (range 85-360 minutes). Details of muscle relaxant administration are summarized below (Fig. 4).

	Unknown anaesthetic	Group 1	Group 2	Group 3	Group 4
Unknown relaxant (7)	5	2			
Gallamine (3)		1	2		
d-tubocurarine (39)	4	6	29		
Alcuronium (29)	2	8	5	13	1
Pancuronium (83)		4		60	19
Succinylcholine (3 times as drip 17 times intermittantly)	1	10	7	2	

20 respiratory problems occurred with these cases and will be discussed later.

Fig. 4.

DISCUSSION

The first question which should be raised is whether muscle relaxants should be used at all in anephric patients, or whether relaxation should be obtained by other anaesthetic agents. In the literature there are reasons put forward for both of these extreme views. A team working in the University of Vienna (9) has suggested that relaxants should be used, coupled with post-operative ventilation for 12-24 hours, until a good diuresis occurs, with elimination of the drug. They base their work on a study of the elimination of radio-active alcuronium during kidney transplantation. However, Fernandes (10) working at the University Hospital in Copenhagen, presented 100 cases of renal transplantation at the Scandinavian Congress in 1971. These were performed without the use of muscle relaxants under cyclopropane anaesthesia.

Between these two extremes, good results have been reported using 'moderate doses' of all the commonly used muscle relaxants. Here it is thought that both extremes are potentially dangerous; the administration of standard 'normal' doses of muscle relaxants and routine post-operative ventilation is associated with the high risk of pulmonary infection in patients under immuno-suppression therapy. Also, in Leiden, post-transplantation care is provided in a special isolation unit, which does not allow close observation of the patient by the anaesthetist and other personnel trained in long term artificial ventilation, thus making this technique exceptionally risky.

To obtain adequate relaxation using volatile agents, high concentrations must be used, and the toxic effects of the agent become apparent. Bad relaxation may account for the long duration of the operations reported by Fernandes (mean duration 6 hours, maximal 11.5 hours) as well as the choice of anaesthetic agent (cyclopropane), which prevented the use of diathermic coagulation. Deep anaesthesia was responsible for the cardiac arrest also mentioned by these authors in their series of one hundred cases.

Although renal transplantation is the most impressive operation performed, it is not the most dangerous in these anephric patients, since immediate diuresis can be expected and hence elimination of the drugs. Bilateral nephrectomy performed in advance, or emergency gastric or gall-bladder resection in a shocked anephric patient, are far more risky to the patient and present a real challenge even to an experienced anaesthetist.

Then the next question – is the choice of anaesthetic technique important in influencing the dose and duration of action of the muscle relaxant used? Recent reports (11, 12) suggest that this is so, and this was the reason for the introduction of methoxyflurane into the technique for this group of patients two years ago. As more experience was obtained it became apparent that the amount of pancuronium bromide required does not alter significantly in groups 1, 3 or 4. Because of this observation combined with the better metabolic effects of neurolept anaesthesia this latter technique was adopted during the last six months (Fig. 5).

In a group of patients for renal transplantation, receiving diazepam in the premedication, and methoxyflurane during the anaesthesia, there was no change in the amount of muscle relaxant used – expressed in micrograms/ kg/hr. When comparison was made with patients undergoing bilateral nephrectomy, diazepam significantly reduced the dose of muscle relaxant required. The mean dose of pancuronium required in diazepam premedicated patients was 26.2% lower than in those premedicated with atropine alone (Fig. 6). This data agreed with the finding of Feldman (11). However, the respiratory problems in this group were not related to the presence or absence of diazepam in the premedication.

If it is decided to use muscle relaxants in anephric patients, the next question is – which relaxant to use, the dosage and the way of administration? The fact that succinylcholine is inactivated in the blood could make it the drug of choice. However, low levels of pseudocholinesterase have been reported immediately after haemodialysis (13, 14), and although this finding has not been confirmed by other workers, many anaesthetists are not enthusiastic about this drug, because of the very real danger of a Phase II block

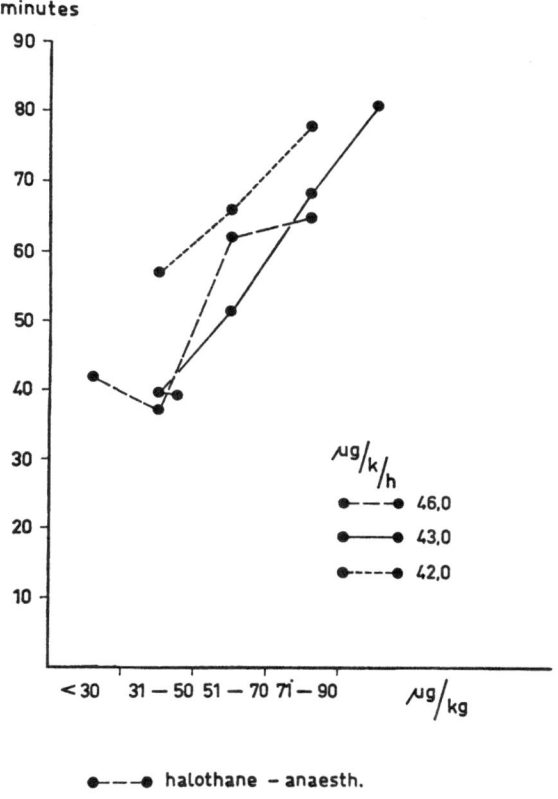

Fig. 5

	With diazepam			No diazepam		
	No. of cases	Mean	S.E.	No. of cases	Mean	S.E.
Transplantations	5	36.4	—	21	36.5	—
Bilat. Nephrect.	24	30.8	± 2.32	15	40.0	± 4.20

t = 6,32
p < 0,01   Fig. 6. Diazepam.

occurring after high doses. During renal transplantation Rolly (4) used a mean dose of 900 mgs of succinylcholine, whilst here in Leiden 750 mgs were used. The rise in serum potassium produced by repeated doses (15) is also a real danger in patients anaesthetised later than 2-3 days post-dialysis.

Used in 20 cases, succinylcholine did not give entire satisfaction. When used intermittantly the relaxation was not good, whilst a continuous infusion necessitated the need for a second intravenous drip, with the associated problems of overhydration (Fig. 7). Post-operatively 5 patients had prolong-

Type anaesthesia	No. of cases	Mean dose (mg/kg/hr)	Respiratory problems	
?	1	?	6	pat. out of 20
I	10	3.8	5	light
II	7	5.3	1	respir. arrest (anaesth.) 5,8 mg/kg/hr) (Pat. 34).
III	2	2.6		
IV	0	—		
Total 20				

Fig. 7. Succinycholine.

ed hypoventilation, with no reversal possible. One patient had a respiratory arrest 30 minutes after the end of the operation. She received 5.8 mg/kg/hr. combined with halothane, nitrous oxide and oxygen, for a renal transplant, and after extubation and apparent adequate ventilation, she had a respiratory arrest during transport and required re-intubation and assisted ventilation for 30 minutes.

The combination of succinylcholine with hexafluorenium has not been studied.

Vandam (16) was the first to mention the tolerance of anephric patients to the non-depolarising blockers. These drugs have the tremendous advantage that their action can be reversed, and also they have been demonstrated to cause less damage to the muscle cells, than the depolarising agents. They do not cause efflux of potassium from the cells, and their duration of action is correlated mainly to redistribution and not to metabolism and elimination (with the exception of gallamine). With d-tubocurare the possibility of biliary elimination has been demonstrated in anephric subjects by Cohen and co-workers (17). Renal elimination can be accounted for completely in terms of glomerular filtration (18) without evoking the additional mechanism of tubular secretion. This is an advantage in kidney transplantation, since in the first post-operative hours, reasonable filtration without improvement in tubular secretion can be expected. All these enumerated advantages would seem to make the non-depolarising drugs the choice for anephric patients.

The next question is which drug to choose? Theoretically the drug should be selected to best fit the length of operation. Morris (19) in 1963 demonstrated that immediately after the administration of d-tubocurare, the highest plasma levels are to be found (Fig. 8). Then a sharp decrease in plasma level

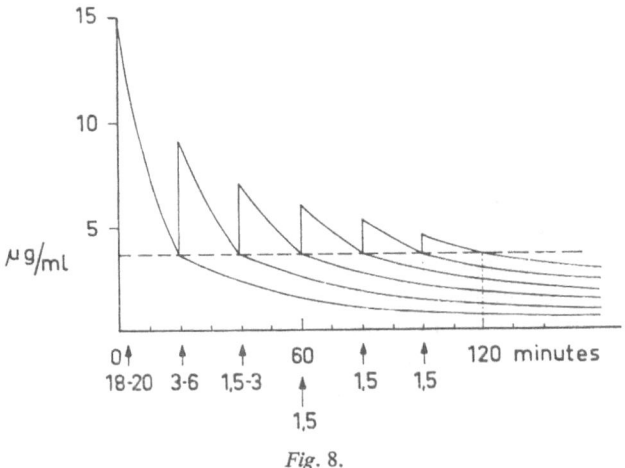

Fig. 8.

follows, followed later by a very gradual decrease over many hours. Incremental doses of the drug are cumulative, and hence the more often incremental doses are given, the higher will be the plasma level at the end of anaesthesia.

Four years later, Paton and Waud put forward the same idea based not on plasma level but on percentage of occupancy of the receptors by the drug (Fig. 9). They demonstrated that only between 70-90% of occupancy can be

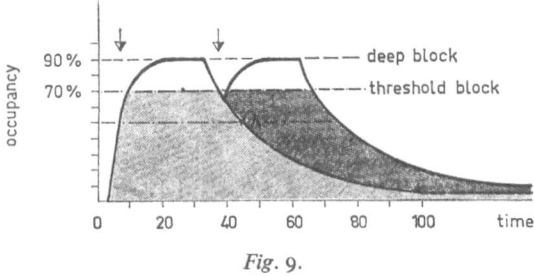

Fig. 9.

shown using nerve stimulators; this small portion being compared to the visible part of the iceberg, the remaining 70% remaining hidden to electrical stimulation. Therefore with 50% occupancy still present, nerve stimulation may show no blockade. This could be highly significant clinically if further injections are made, causing difficult antagonism or residual curarisation.

If this is true for normal patients, it is even more so for anephric ones. The way in which patients with normal kidneys differ from those with inadequate renal function is that the former exhibit no ill effects from residual curarisation since, in addition to redistribution, the plasma level of relaxant (or occupancy) will progressively fall during the post anaesthetic period due to renal excretion. This explains why out of a total of 5,000 relaxant anaesthetics performed here per year, no complications have been observed in patients with good renal function, whilst in the transplantation group 20 complications have been reported.

It was noted that the dosage of pancuronium calculated with reference to the surface area of the patient, did not correlate any better with the duration of action of the drug, than by basing the dose on the weight of the subject. Therefore, it was decided to base the dosage on body weight using the correction of Foldes.

Corrected body weight = measured body weight + (35 – *measured body weight*). This has the advantage that the data is readily available and is less alien to clinical anaesthetists.

Out of the three patients who received gallamine triethiode, two had ventilation problems.

One had to be ventilated for 12 hours post-operatively (patient 102). He had received 740 µg/kg/hr. of relaxant combined with ether and halothane.

The second case (patient 93) had a 'difficult' post anaesthetic period – no further data is available. These results agree with previous experience of other workers.

The good results obtained with gallamine by White and his colleagues from California, published in 1971, can be explained by the very low dosage of drug used – mean 445 µg/kg/hr with many cases receiving under 300 µg/kg/hr. Anaesthesia was maintained in most of their cases with halothane, latterly with neurolept anaesthesia.

From the 39 cases to whom d-tubocurare was administered, 4 cases were associated with an unknown anaesthetic sequence and 29 with ether – halothane and nitrous oxide (Fig. 10). A mean dose of 117 µg/kg/hr. was given ± 14.74 (S.D.) ± 3.345 (S.E.M.) with a range of 40-280. This data confirms the wide range of sensitivity to d-tubocurare, as reported in the literature. There were two post-operative ventilation problems – patients 8 and 84. Patient 8 received a very high total dose of drug (280 µg/kg/hr.) and also re-

Anaesthesia		With II		
?	4	117 ± 14,7 µg/kg/hr		
I	6	40 — 280 range		
II	29	Difficulties:		
III	—	Pat. 8	280 µg	8 reinj./2h30
IV	—	Pat. 84	116 µg	7 reinj.
Total	39			

Fig. 10. d-Tubocurarine.

ceived this dosage through a large number of injections (8 in 2 hr. 30 min.). Patient 84 received a low total dose (106 µgrams/kg/hr.) but also received a large number of injections.

Alcuronium was used in 29 cases, the mean dose administered being 116 µgrams/kg/hr. with halothane (Fig. 11). 131 with ether-halothane; 160 with

Type anaesthesia	No. of patients	Mean dose (µg/kg/hr)	S.D.	Problem patients	
?	2	?		With II	
I	8	116	± 13.5	Pat. 44 – 190 µg	5 reinj./1h40
II	5	131	± 15.4	Pat. 57 – 160 µg	7 reinj./2h
III	13	106	± 11.3	Pat. 91 – 170 µg	14 reinj./4h
IV	1	98	—		
Total	29				

Fig. 11. Alcuronium.

methoxyflurane; and 98 with neurolept analgesia (one patient). Three problems occurred in the post-operative period, all in patients who had received ether-halothane nitrous oxide anaesthesia. All the cases received high total doses, and all had multiple injections of relaxant. The 'problem patients' in the d-tubocurare and alcuronium series demonstrate the fact that the more times a re-injection of relaxant occurs, the greater the possibility of residual curarisation occurring in that case, with difficult antagonism and recurarisation. Thus a large initial dose of drug is better than many smaller ones.

Pancuronium bromide was administered 83 times to 56 patients in this series, and was the most studied relaxant used in anephric patients. It was administered 4 times in combination with halothane, 60 times with methoxyflurane and 19 times with neurolept anaesthesia (Fig. 12).

'Problems' occurred in 8 patients.

Type anaesthesia	No. of patients	Mean dose (μg/kg/hr)		Problem patients		Remarks
				Mean dose	Last dose	
I	4	46	Pat. 59	52	30′ ⎫	Reint.
			Pat. 38	51	20′ ⎬	extra
III	60	43	Pat. 103	52	30′ ⎭	neo.
			Pat. 31	46	100′	Acidosys
IV	19	42	Pat. 32	52	120′ ⎫	
			Pat. 74	38	15′ ⎬	Self com-
			Pat. 82	94	30′ ⎭	plaint
			Pat. 100	53	90′	
Total	83					

Fig. 12. Pancuronium.

One was an obvious recurarisation (patient 59) requiring immediate intubation, a further dose of neostigmine and ventilation with pure oxygen for half an hour. The cause was a high total dose of drug (52 μg/kg/hr.) plus a short interval between the final dose and the end of the operation (30 minutes).

Two patients were asleep at the end of the operation and had clinically depressed ventilation which responded well to an additional dose of neostigmine (patients 38 and 103).

One patient had depressed ventilation due to severe acidosis. Correction of this with sodium bicarbonate resulted in adequate ventilation being established with return of consciousness (patient 33).

The other four 'problem' patients were wide awake and complaining about 'difficulty in breathing'. Additional doses of neostigmine returned their breathing to normal (patients 32, 74, 82 and 100).

If we exclude from this series the acidotic patient and the four awake ones whose only complaint was subjective difficulty in breathing, the three respiratory depressions occurring in 83 pancuronium administrations represent the lowest percentage of ventilation problems observed with the various muscle relaxants used in Leiden.

Pancuronium has the advantage of maintaining cardiac output (21), which makes it the drug of choice in anaemic, hypovolaemic patients. Since only two or, occasionally, three injections of drug are necessary for a 2-3 hour procedure, the problems of accumulation are less. The main problem with this drug (as with other relaxants) is that the range of individual sensitivity is large, and no clinical dose-duration relationship can be found in patients with diminished renal function. This agrees with the data of Orth (22) obtained in patients with normal renal function. In consequence no 'standard' can be recommended (Fig. 13).

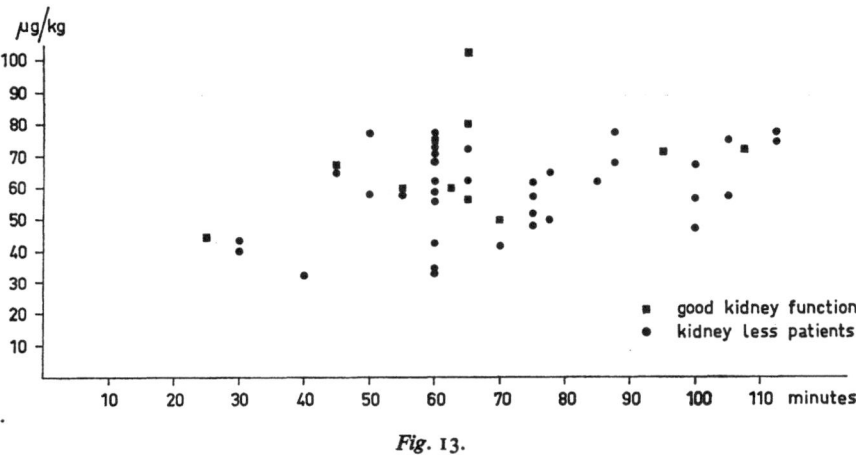

Fig. 13.

Do additional factors play a part in the dose duration of these drugs, or in the incidence of 'ventilation problems' in anephric patients? It is thought so, but some of these factors remain unclear. In this series, the level of serum potassium does not appear to affect the duration of muscle relaxation. Patients with low potassium (3.1-3.2 mEq/l) tolerated the same dose of relaxant as those with very high potassium (5.9-6.6 mEq/l).

The presence of diazepam in premedication reduces the amount of relaxant required as mentioned above.

The circulatory condition of the patient is very important (Fig. 14). Two patients received pancuronium on two occasions, the first whilst normovo-

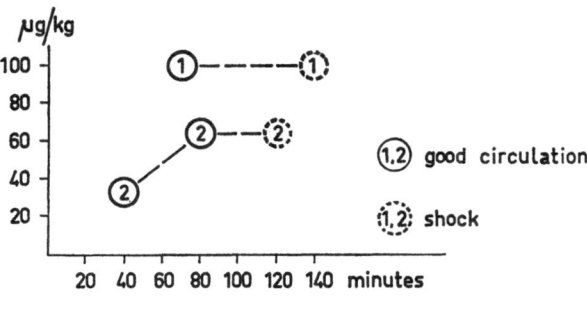

Fig. 14.

laemic and the latter during hemorrhagic shock. In shock the same amount of drug caused paralysis for $1\frac{1}{2}$ times as long in one case, twice as long in the other.

It has become apparent from this study that the experience of the anaesthetist is important (Fig. 15). Ten different anaesthetists administered pan-

Anaesthesist	Cases
I	1 **2** 3 4 **5** 6 7 **8** 9 10 11 13 16 19 20 22 27 28 29 30
	31 32 34 35 36 39 40 41 42 43 47 49 54 60
II	12 17 18 24
III	**14** 23 55
IV	**15** 21 59
V	25
VI	26 **38**
VII	33 45 48 52 57
VIII	37 50
IX	**44** 46 51 56 58
X	**53**

Fig. 15. Bold numbers represent 'problem patients'.

curonium bromide to anephric patients, and all 'problem patients' occurred with anaesthetists dealing with their first dialysis patients.

Another important factor is the time between the last dose of drug and the end of the operation (Fig. 16). Cases 38, 59, 74, 82 and 103 illustrate this

Case no.	Total dose (μg/kg/hr)	Interval		Remarks
		Last dose of drug	End of the operation	
59	52		30'	Reint.
31	46		100'	*Acidosis*
32	52		120'	Awake
38	51		20'	
74	38		*15'*	⎫
82	94		30'	⎬ Awake
100	53		90'	⎭
103	52		30'	

Fig. 16.

point. They all presented 'problems' and all received the last dose of drug quite near the conclusion of the procedure (15-30 mins.). These patients were also amongst the first anephric cases of the anaesthetists, showing that a more experienced person is better able to judge the length of operation and thus able to ensure that smaller doses of relaxants are used, and the final one is given well before the end of anaesthesia.

Acidosis prolongs the effect of pancuronium. Patient 31 received an average amount of relaxant with optimal timing of the injections. Despite this his ventilation was depressed. This returned to normal after correction of his acidosis with sodium bicarbonate.

CONCLUSION

From the experience of the anaesthetic department in Leiden, muscle relaxants need to be given to anephric patients for major intra abdominal surgery. Because the range of sensitivity to the drug is so wide, care must be taken to keep the dose as low as possible. Non-depolarising drugs gave better results than succinylcholine, and from this series, the longer lasting agents (d-tubocurarine, and pancuronium) are indicated since fewer incremental doses are required. Premedication with diazepam prolongs their action, as does shock or acidosis.

The use of small, repeated doses should be abandoned in favour of an adequate initial dose, followed by smaller amounts when required – not too near the completion of the operation. Because of this, the experienced anaesthetist has better results. Thus modern surgery is a serious team work between surgeon and anaesthetist, and not the 'brilliant demonstration of one man's skill'.

REFERENCES

1. Feldman, S. A. & Tyrell, M. F., A new theory of the action of muscle relaxants. Proc· Anaesth. Res. Soc. *Brit. J. Anaesth.* 42, 1, 91 (1970).
2. Waser, P. G., Eine molekulare Theorie zur Wirkungsweise curarisierender Stoffe. *Anaesthesist.* 20, 1, 23 (1971).
3. Hannington-Kiff, J. G., Residual postoperative paralysis. *Proc. roy. Soc. Med.* 63, 1, 73 (1970).
4. Rolly, G., Anaesthesia for renal transplantation. *Anaesthesist* 18, 8, 270 (1970).
5. Samuel, J. R. & Powell, D., Renal transplantation. Anaesthetic experiences with 100 cases. *Anaesthesia* 25, 2, 165 (1970).
6. White, R. D., De Weerd, J. H. & Dawson, B., Gallamine in anaesthesia for patients with chronic renal failure undergoing bilateral nephrectomy. *Anesth. Analg. (Curr.) Res.* 50, 1, 11 (1971).
7. Singer, M. M., Dutton, R. & Way, W. L., Untoward results of gallamine administration during bilateral nephrectomy. *Brit. J. Anaesth.* 43, 4, 404 (1971).
8. Popescu, D. T., Boeré, L. A. & Houwing, A. H. J., Methoxyflurane anaesthesia in kidney transplantation. *European Congress of Anaesthesiology*, Prague 1970.
9. Höfer, R., Krenn, J., Pfeiffer, G. & Steinbezeithner, M., Untersuchungen zur Ausscheidung von d-allylnor-toxiferin bei Niertransplantation. *Anaesthesist* 18, 9, 304 (1969).

10. Fernandes, A. I. & Hansen, D. D., Anaesthesia for 100 cases of kidney transplantation. Communication. 10th Scandinavian Society of Anaesthesiology, Lund 1971.
11. Feldman, S. A. & Crawley, B. E., Interaction of diazepam with the muscle relaxant drugs. *Brit. med. J.* 2, 336 (1970).
12. Walts, L. F. & Dillon, J. B., The influence of the anaesthetic agent in the action of curare in man. *Anesth. Analg. Curr. Res.* 49, 1, 27 (1970).
13. Thomas, J. L. & Holmes, J. A., Plasma cholinesterase levels in dialysis patients. *Anaesth. Analg. Curr. Res.* 49, 2, 323 (1970).
14. Virtue, R. W., Chapter 9 in Starzl Th. J., *Experience in renal transplantation.* Philadelphia (Pa.) 1964.
15. Weintraub, H. D. and coll., Changes in plasma potassium concentrations after depolarizing blockers in anaesthetised man. *Brit. J. Anaesth.* 41, 12, 1048 (1969).
16. Vandam, L. D. and coll., Anaesthetic aspects of renal homotransplantation in man. *Anesthesiology* 23, 6, 783 (1962).
17. Cohen, E. N., Brewer, H. W. & Smith, D., The metabolism and elimination of muscle relaxants. In: *Scientific foundation of anaesthesia*, chapter 4. Scurr, C. & Feldman, S. A. (eds.) London 1970.
18. Morris, L. E., Plasma levels of d-tubocurarine. *Brit. J. Anaesth.* 35, 1, 35 (1963).
19. Paton, W. D. M. & Waud, D. R., The margin of safety of neuro-muscular transmission. *J. Physiol.* 191, 1, 59 (1967).
20. Kelman, G. R. & Kennedy, B. R., Cardiovascular effects of pancuronium in man. *Brit. J. Anaesth.* 43, 4, 335 (1971).
21. Van Orth, P., Klinische ervaringen met het nieuwe spierrelaxant pancuronium bromide. *Ned. T. Geneesk.* 115, 8, 316 (1971).

PART THREE

EFFECTS AND SIDE-EFFECTS
OF ANAESTHETIC AGENTS

THE TRUTH ABOUT ANTIHYPERTENSIVE AND ANAESTHETIC DRUGS

L. STAMENKOVIC

In 1968 it was estimated that 15 million people living in the United States were hypertensive. Five million of these were receiving antihypertensive therapy, most of them in combination with diuretics (1). Because of the variety of agents used and the little data available on the combined effects of the drugs, makes categorisation and analysis of their effects is very complicated and difficult. The anaesthetist is not an uninterested bystander, he actively participates in the everyday struggle for the life of the hypertensive patient.

Whether treated or not, these patients require careful individual assessment several days before an anaesthetic is planned. The origin, the severity and especially secondary forms of hypertension must be detected. Some of the causes of secondary hypertension may be amenable to surgery – for instance obstruction of the blood flow to the kidney in renal parenchymal compression, renal artery disease or compression, primary hyperaldosteronism caused by a tumour of the adrenal cortex, phaeochromocytoma, Cushing's syndrome in cases with pituitary tumour and adrenal hyperplasia, coarctation of the aorta, etc. Therefore, an adequate history, joint consultation with a physician or cardiologist, detailed examination of the cardiovascular system, ECG, X-rays of the chest and abdomen, serum electrolytes, blood sugar and urine analysis, are all essential in the pre-operative examination of the patient. Opthalmoscopy provides the best objective assessment of the degree of arteriosclerosis. Arteriosclerotic disease involving kidneys, central nervous system, and heart, or the presence of an unsuspected phaeochromocytoma, uncontrolled severe or malignant hypertension all may prove very dangerous in association with anaesthesia. Also dangerous is the presence of potent or unknown antihypertensive therapy.

Autoregulation of blood flow in the elderly arteriosclerotic hypertensive patient may be seriously impaired, and ischemia to the vital organs, heart, brain and kidneys, may occur during hypotensive periods (2).

The pre-operative assessment of the patient's response to anaesthesia by vascular and baroreflex activity is unlikely to be of value, and is of academic interest only (3).

Evidence of left ventricular failure, provided by gallop rhythm, history of orthopnoea or paroxysmal nocturnal dyspnoea (cardiac asthma) is a contra-indication to immediate anaesthesia, and treatment with digitalis, diuretics and antihypertensive agents should be instituted (3).

Patients who are receiving treatment for mild to moderate hypertension should discontinue their antihypertensive therapy for several days prior to elective surgery (4). Usually their blood pressure will remain normal for the next few weeks. Hospital environment and bed rest have well known hypotensive effects, and general and spinal anaesthesia will result in further hypotension which may continue during convalescence (5).

Untreated hypertension constitutes a serious risk to patients undergoing anaesthesia and surgery. Withdrawal of their antihypertensive therapy before anaesthesia is potentially dangerous both during the pre-operative period and also during anaesthesia. The high incidence of myocardial ischemia occurring during anaesthesia in untreated symptom-free hypertensive patients, would suggest that treatment is recommended before anaesthesia and surgery (3).

The presence of high blood pressure is significant only when it is related to age, sex, family history, symptoms, signs and function. Organic effects of

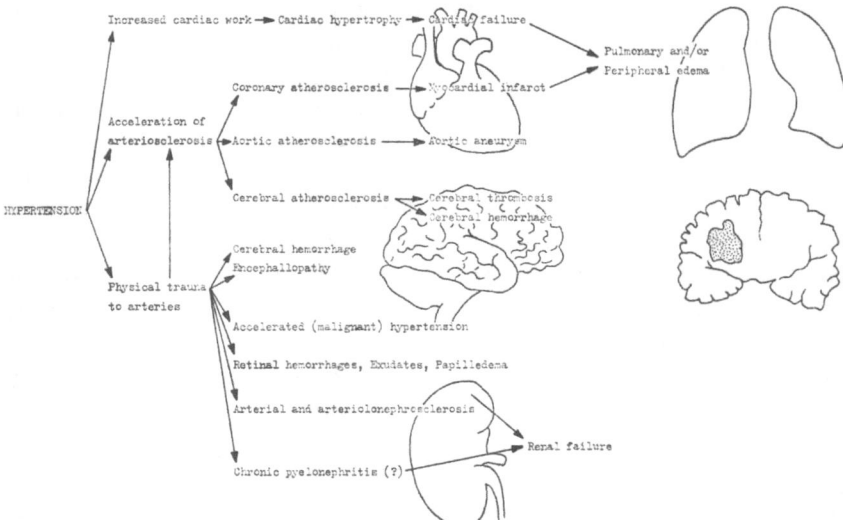

Fig. 1. Organic effects of hypertension.

hypertension are indications for drug therapy, which should reduce blood pressure by several mechanisms:

1. Decrease peripheral resistance.
2. Reduce cardiac output.
3. Volume depletion (extracellular, intravascular or both).

MECHANISMS OF HYPERTENSION

Established untreated essential hypertension is characterized by a raised systemic vascular resistance, with a normal or slightly sub-normal cardiac output (6). It can be separated into three aetiological causes: neurogenic, humoral and anatomical. These do not operate separately, and hence blood pressure, vascular resistance and tissue perfusion result from an equilibrium between the many mechanisms (7, 8). The fundamental deficit appears to be the presence of hyper-reactive smooth muscle in the arterioles (9).

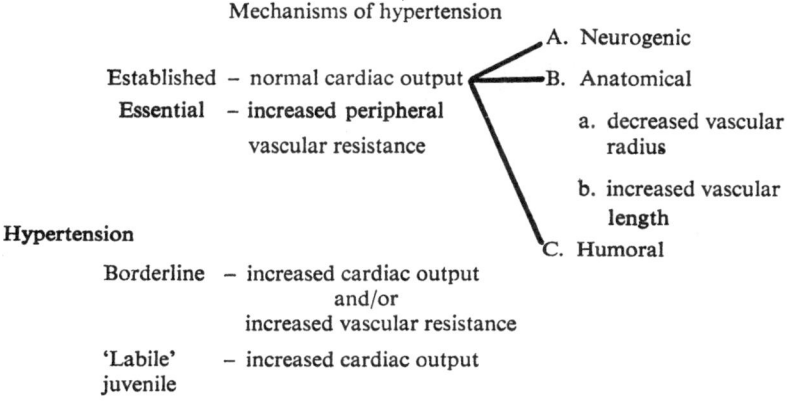

Fig. 2.

'Labile' hypertension in young patients is predominantly due to an elevated cardiac output (10, 11, 12), although this early hyperdynamic state may develop into essential hypertension with raised systemic vascular resistance.

In cases of borderline hypertension, these patients have an increased cardiac output with 'normal' peripheral resistance in the recumbent position. Blood pressure is maintained at a higher level but in a way closely resembling that in normotensive subjects, whether the cardiac output is high or low and resistance normal or elevated. Consequently borderline hypertension is not caused solely by an increased cardiac output.

Cardiac output and peripheral resistance are dependant on the tone in the peripheral blood vessels (Fig. 3). Blockade of vasoconstrictor fibres passing

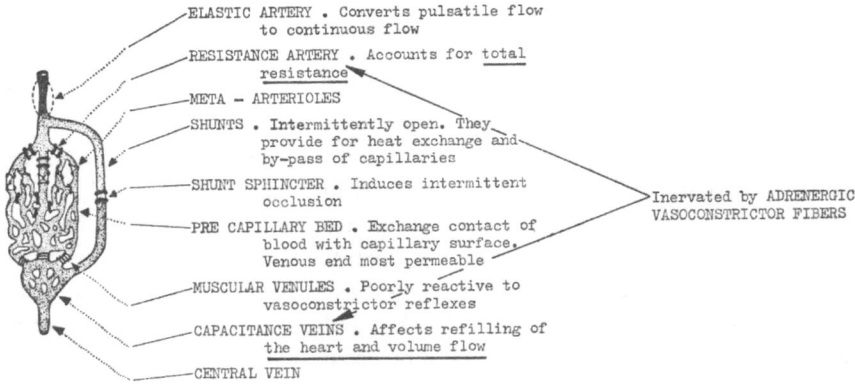

Fig. 3. Functional classification of vascular segments.

to resistance vessels, will lower the peripheral resistance, and blockade of fibres passing to capacitance veins will induce vasodilatation with reduction in venous return, and hence cardiac output. These are the main principles involved in antihypertensive therapy.

Both resistance and capacitance vessels are innervated by adrenergic vasoconstrictor fibres. Normally the blood volume is distributed so that the capillary bed contains 5-7.5% and the venous bed 60-75%. As a loss of venous tone may increase its capacity by two and a half times, it is easy to understand the dependence of central venous pressure and heart refilling on the capacitance veins. The actual level of blood pressure is a problem to the anaesthetist as well as the nature of the antihypertensive agent used.

VASOMOTOR CENTRE DEPRESSING AGENTS

Veratrum alkaloids inhibit the vasomotor centre and stimulate the vagal nucleus. This results in peripheral vasodilatation, bradycardia and hypotension. The bradycardia can be abolished, but the blood pressure only partially restored by atropine.

GANGLIONIC BLOCKING AGENTS

These powerful drugs block both sympathetic and parasympathetic ganglia. Their effect on blood pressure is more pronounced in the erect position. Part of their hypotensive action is due to the direct action on smooth muscle, causing relaxation, and also histamine release. The intravenous use of these drugs in emergencies or for hypotensive anaesthesia (trimetaphan Arfonad) must be very cautious as there are other effects apart from the ganglionic blockade.

ADRENERGIC BLOCKING AGENTS (FIG. 4)

Rauwolfia alkaloids, reserpine and serpasil, block the uptake and transfer

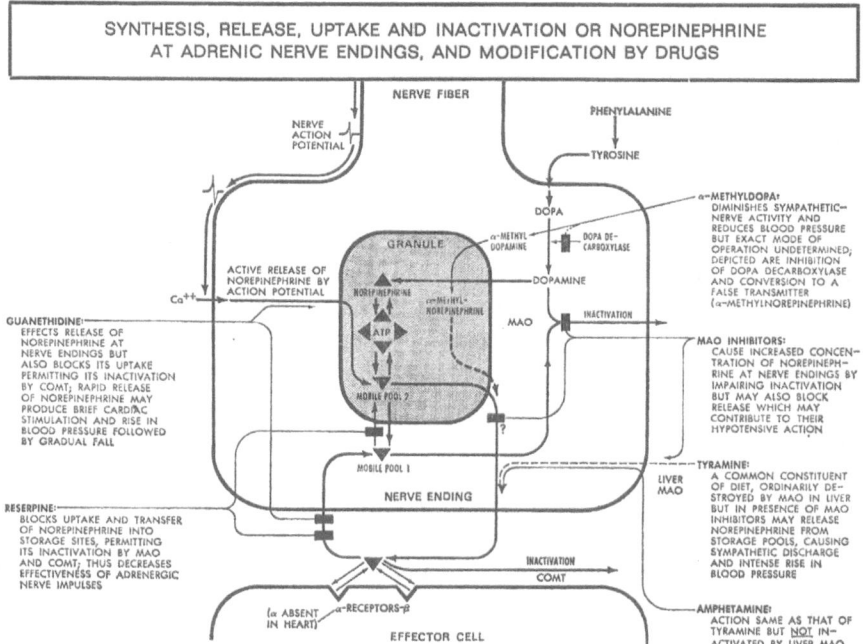

Fig. 4. From: The CIBA Collection of Medical Illustrations. Vol. 5 Heart. section II, plate 84.

of noradrenaline into the storage sites: the brain, blood vessels, adrenal medulla and sympathetic ganglionic fibres, and hence permit its inactivation by MAO. So the decrease in the effectiveness of cardiac adrenergic nerve impulses may result in bradycardia, decreased cardiac output, lowered blood pressure and impairment of the sympathetic component of compensatory cardiovascular reflexes. Their action may continue for 10-20 days after withdrawal of the drug. Problems caused by the depletion of catecholamines may be treated by the prompt correction of fluid loss, atropine, and appropriate pressor agents, thus avoiding the need to discontinue these drugs several weeks before the operation. Reserpine may induce heart block in digitalised patients.

Central depletion of noradrenaline reduces halothane requirements during anaesthesia, and also reduces the normal response to hypovolaemia. Hence hypotension may result and increased neurovascular lability. Common complications of reserpine therapy are: aggravation of asthma by bronchiolar constriction and secretion, peptic ulcer, suicidal depression and nasal congestion. This latter complication may cause feeding difficulties in a neonate whose mother has received reserpine.

Guanethidine (Ismelin) impairs the release and uptake of noradrenaline from its storage site at peripheral adrenergic nerve endings, thus permitting its inactivation. If given rapidly or in high dosage it may briefly produce cardiac stimulation and a rise in blood pressure due to the rapid release of stored noradrenaline.

Cardiovascular reflexes which are dependant upon the sympathetic nervous system are greatly depressed, and postural hypotension and a reduction in cardiac output are common. In patients with myocardial or renal insufficiency guanethidine must be very carefully employed. At the final sympathetic effector site, guanethidine produces pharmacological hypersensitivity to adrenaline, noradrenaline and all sympathomimetics which act directly on the receptor. This results in the effects of these drugs on the heart being grossly exaggerated. The effects of guanethidine persist for 3 to 4 days after cessation of therapy, and halothane requirements for anaesthesia are not affected.

Alpha-methyldopa (Aldomet) also depletes catecholamine stores in the central nervous system, peripheral tissues and nerves. It inhibits decarboxylase, which is necessary for noradrenaline synthesis, and is itself converted to alpha-methyl noradrenaline which is physiologically less effective than noradrenaline, and may replace it at the nerve terminals (14). These effects are much less important than with the rauwolfia alkaloids or guanethidine, because the adrenergic nerves act normally, and the excretion of catecholamine metabolites can be demonstrated, even when hypotensive doses of aldomet are used (15). Consequently it is wise to stop reserpine or guanethidine before an operation, substituting methyldopa which stays in the body for only 24 hours.

MONOAMINE OXIDASE INHIBITOR (MAOI)
Monoamine oxidase inhibitors impair the inactivation of noradrenaline, and

hence in the presence of these drugs the concentration of noradrenaline in the storage granules and nerve endings is increased. Thus, drugs which indirectly cause the release of noradrenaline from peripheral nerve endings, for instance, amphetamine and tyramine, may cause a greatly exaggerated sympathetic discharge. In the presence of MAOI there may be a hypertensive crisis, which can be very dramatic or even fatal, after the consumption of tyramine containing substances (e.g. cheese, wine, broad beans, meat and yeast extracts). If the stores of noradrenaline are so increased, the use of an indirectly acting pressor amine (depending on the body's store of catecholamines) may result in a dangerously potentiated pressor response (16). Examples of the indirectly acting amines are ephedrine, methamphetamine and mephentermine. Directly acting pressor amines, such as noradrenaline (Levophed), adrenaline, methoxamine hydrochloride (Vasoxyl), phenylephrine (Neosynephrine) and metaraminol (Aramine) (17) are safer, but noradrenaline may also be potentiated.

MAO inhibitors increase the effects of barbiturates, morphine, pethidine, anaesthetic agents and insulin. Pargyline remains effective for 9 days, and whenever possible, this drug should be discontinued 3-4 weeks before operation.

ALPHA RECEPTOR BLOCKING AGENTS
These cause dilatation of the resistance vessels of the peripheral vascular bed including the vessels of striated muscle. There are no important alpha receptors in the heart since the heart contains essentially only beta receptors. Alpha blockers have no direct effect on the myocardium nor can they block reflex sympathetic activity, or alter the effects of sympathomimetic drugs on the heart. Because of their systemic action (a fall in blood pressure) a reflex tachycardia may result.

BETA RECEPTOR BLOCKING AGENTS
Propranolol (Inderal) augments the action of depolarising and reduces the action of non-depolarising muscle relaxants.

DIRECT SMOOTH MUSCLE INHIBITOR
Hydralazine (Apresoline) has a direct action on vascular smooth muscle. Its side effects include an increased cardiac output, angina, headache, palpitations and nervousness. An increase in renal blood flow results. After an oral dose, the duration of action of the drug is less than 12 hours.

DIURETICS

Diuretics such as chlorothiazide (Diural), hydrochlorothiazide (Esidrex), chlorothalidone (Hygroton) and ethacrinic acid, all reduce peripheral resistance, and have a hypotensive action, potentiating more potent antihypertensive drugs (17) (Fig. 5). The most important hazard of thiazide therapy is

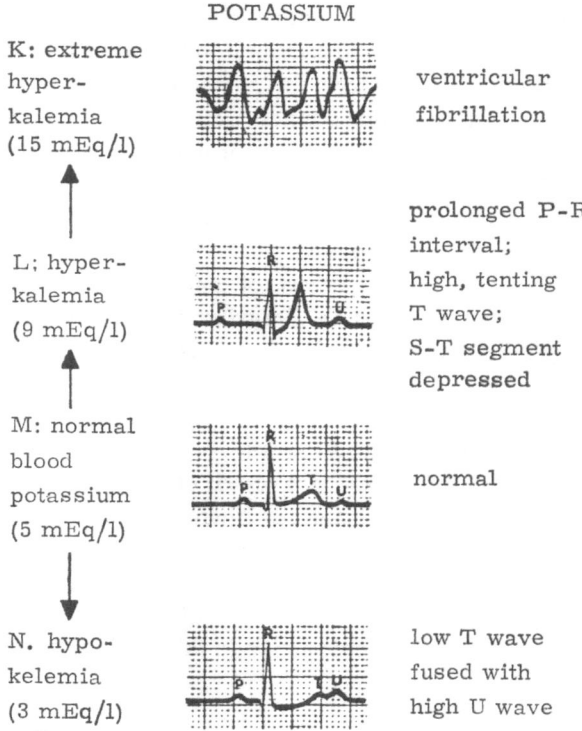

POTASSIUM

K: extreme hyper-kalemia (15 mEq/l) — ventricular fibrillation

L; hyper-kalemia (9 mEq/l) — prolonged P-R interval; high, tenting T wave; S-T segment depressed

M: normal blood potassium (5 mEq/l) — normal

N. hypo-kelemia (3 mEq/l) — low T wave fused with high U wave

Fig. 5. Hazards of hypokalaemia induced by diuretics.

potassium depletion. This may result in cardiac arrhythmias particularly in patients receiving digitalis. This results in defects in cardiac condition precipitating digitalis toxicity. Increased sensitivity to the non-depolarising muscle relaxants (e.g. d-tubocurarine) occurs in hypokalaemia due to impaired neuromuscular function. Also paralytic ileus may occur. Thiazide diuretics often produce hypokalaemia with hypochloremic alkalosis. With combination, assessment of the degree of potassium depletion may be difficult, because the serum potassium level may remain normal despite intracellular hypokalaemia due to a shift of the potassium from the cells into the plasma. If urine output is adequate, potassium chloride may be given intravenously in a concentration not greater than 60 mEq/l, and at a rate not exceeding 20 mEq/hr., monitoring the serum potassium and watching the electrocardiogram.

INDUCTION AGENTS

Thiopentone (Pentothal) causes arterial hypotension in normotensive subjects. This occurs as a result of a reduction in cardiac output (18, 19) and therefore it should be injected very slowly (20) giving the smallest possible sleep dose in a 2.5% solution.

Diazepam (Valium) and Propanidid (Epontol) can cause dramatic but transient hypotension in hypertensive patients.

Methohexitone (Brevital) produces a more profound hypotension than thiopentone in hypertensive patients. This is unlike its effect in normotensive ones. Neurolept analgesia induced with a combination of droperidol and fentanyl appeared to offer protection to the electrocardiographic and haemodynamic responses to induction of anaesthesia, laryngoscopy and endotracheal intubation in untreated hypertensive patients. Also less hypotension resulted in patients receiving antihypertensive therapy. It offers marginally more protection than other agents against hypertension, tachycardia, and dysrhythmias associated with laryngoscopy and tracheal intubation (21).

Induction of anaesthesia is potentially the most dangerous period since sudden hypotension may lead to bradycardia and myocardial ischemia.

CIRCULATORY RESPONSES TO LARYNGOSCOPY AND TRACHEAL INTUBATION

Following mechanical stimulation of the upper respiratory tract, the nose, the epipharynx, the laryngopharynx and the tracheobronchial tree (22) or after aspiration of secretions from the trachea, in patients both with normal cardiovascular reflexes (23) or exaggerated ones due to autonomic overactivity (24), in man the predominant cardiovascular response is tachycardia (Fig. 6). Arterial hypertension results from the increased cardiac output rather than an increase in systemic vascular resistance, and is associated with a transient rise in central venous pressure (24) and enhanced neuronal activity in the cervical sympathetic fibres. These cardiovascular responses are most pronounced during stimulation of the epipharynx (22, 23). Laryngoscopy with the Macintosh blade, because it compresses the soft tissues of

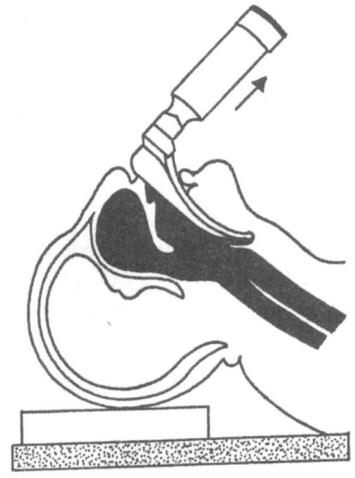

Tachycardia

Increased cardiac output

Arterial hypertension

Rise in central venous pressure

Enhanced neuronal activity in cervical
sympathetic efferent fibers

Fig. 6. Cardiovascular responses on mechanical stimulation of the upper respiratory tract.

the anterior epipharynx, produced a significantly greater hypertensive response than the straight bladed Wis-Foregger laryngoscope (25). Blind nasal intubation produces no significant increase in systolic or mean arterial pressure, nor of heart rate in comparison to the response to laryngoscopy in the same patient.

Once the endotracheal tube has been inserted and the laryngoscope withdrawn, the hypertension and sinus tachycardia quickly subsides, but arrhythmias may persist for a few minutes. These usually take the form of premature ventricular contractions or ventricular bigeminy. Bradycardia, in response to laryngoscopy and intubation is rare. In both treated and untreated hypertensive patients these cardiovascular reflexes are more pronounced, because these patients are prone to greater changes in arterial pressure. It would appear rational to prevent these responses by the prophylactic use of beta-adrenergic blocking agents.

CARDIOVASCULAR EFFECTS OF ANAESTHESIA

The reduction of stroke volume and cardiac output ocurring during halothane anaesthesia, is due to depression of myocardial contractility (26, 27). Thus the site of depression lies within the muscle cell rather than in the autonomic post ganglionic nerves or the adrenergic receptors (28).

The ejection of blood from the left ventricle is influenced by the amount of resistance and impedance of the arterial tree (26, 29). The stroke volume of the depressed heart is especially reduced if the resistance to ejection is increased, and increased when the resistance falls (27).

The high systemic vascular resistance found in hypertensive patients should not remain unaltered during anaesthesia. This would mean an increased load on the depressed ventricular muscle, resulting in left ventricular failure, with an elevated end-diastolic pressure in the left ventricle. Myocardial ischemia is evident from the appearance of marked ST and T wave depressions associated with a low mean arterial pressure ($<$ 50% of the awake MAP) (3).

This has been demonstrated in dogs anaesthetised with halothane, a high systemic vascular resistance being produced with phenylephine (27). Therefore, if peripherally acting pressor agents are used at all, they should be used in great caution during anaesthesia in patients with hypertension. During halothane anaesthesia, severe arrhythmias may occur in untreated hypertensive patients and those treated with reserpine. These disappear when the halothane is withdrawn.

If hypertensive patients are well controlled prior to anaesthesia, they behave similarly to normotensive ones during anaesthesia. Their cardiac output drops to the same extent (30% approx.) (3), due to a reduction of both heart rate and stroke volume. In untreated or inadequately controlled hypertensive patients, the great fall in the mean arterial pressure is due to a reduction of the high systemic vascular resistance. Therefore antihypertensive therapy should not be stopped before anaesthesia, unless there is a compelling reason. Careful balance of electrolytes and circulating blood volume, detailed information about the type, dose and last administration of antihypertensive drug are mandatory prior to anaesthesia.

NEUROLEPT ANAESTHESIA
Since the heart contains essentially only beta receptors, the alpha blocking effect of droperidol has no direct action on the myocardium. Neither can it block reflex sympathetic activity. Droperidol blocks the pressor response to adrenaline but not to noradrenaline. The inotropic and chronotropic effects of catecholamines on the heart remain intact.

If we consider the electrocardiographic and haemodynamic responses to induction of anaesthesia, laryngoscopy and endotracheal intubation, operation, intra-operative bleeding and recovery then neurolept anaesthesia produces less arterial hypotension than any other type of anaesthesia in treated or untreated hypertensive patients. Established alpha adrenergic blockade, exhibits a linear response to the loss and replacement of circulating blood volume. Therefore it is necessary to maintain a physiological circulating volume from the beginning, the best guide being the maintenance of the central venous pressure at about 10 cm H_2O. The dilated microcirculation plus the adequate circulating volume will support tissue perfusion, with cardiovascular stability.

Further investigation of neurolept anaesthesia and recovery from the same in hypertensive patients is under way.

REFERENCES

1. Palmer, F. R., Antihypertensive agents. *International Anaesthesiology Clinics* 6, 1, 131 (1968).
2. Hikler, R. B. & Vandam, L. D., Hypertension. *Anaesthesiology* 33, 214 (1970).
3. Prys-Roberts, C., Meloche, R. & Foëx, P., Cardiovascular responses of treated and untreated patients. *Brit. J. Anaesth.* (1971).
4. Thurm, R. H. & Smith, W. M., On resetting of 'Barostats' in hypertensive patients. *J. Amer. med. Ass.* 201, 301 (1967).
5. Breslin, J. D. & Swinton, W. N., Elective surgery in hypertensive patients – pre-operative considerations. *Surg. Clin. N. Amer.* 50, 3, 585 (1970).
6. Werkö, L. & Lagerlöf, H., Studies on the circulation in man. IV: Cardiac output and blood pressure in the right auricle, right ventricle and pulmonary artery in patients with hypertensive cardiovascular disease. *Acta med. scand.* 133, 427; 1949.
7. Page, I. H. & McCubbin, J. W., Physiology of arterial hypertension. *Handbook of Physiology, Section 2, Circulation*, Vol. 3. Washington (D.C.) 1966.
8. Page, I. H., The mosaic theory of arterial hypertension, its interpretation. *Perspect. Biol. Med.* 10, 325 (1967).
9. Doyle, S. E. & Fraser, J. R. E., Essential hypertension and inheritance of vascular reactivity. *Lancet* 2, 509 (1961).
10. Eich, R. H., Cuddy, R. P., Smulyan, H. & Lyons, R. H., Hemodynamics in labile hypertension: a follow-up study. *Circulation* 34, 299 (1966).
11. Frolich, E. D., Tarazi, R. C. & Dustan, H. P., Re-examination of the hemodynamics of hypertension. *Amer. J. med. Sci.* 257, 9 (1969).
12. Sannerstedt, R., Hemodynamic findings at rest and during exercise in mild arterial hypertension. *Amer. J. med. Sci.* 258, 70 (1969).
13. Gregerson, M. I. & Rawson, R. A., Blood volume. *Physiol. Rev.* 39, 307 (1959).
14. Day, M. D. & Rand, M. J., A hypothesis for the mode of action of alpha methyldopa in relieving hypertension. *J. Pharm. Pharmacol.* 15, 221-224 (1963).
15. Nickerson, M., Drugs inhibiting adrenergic nerves and structures innervated by them. In: Goodman, L. S. & Gilman, A. (eds.), *The pharmacological basis of therapeutics.* p. 716-735, New York 1965.
16. Stark, D. C. C., Letters: Effects of giving vasopressors to patients on monoamino-oxidase inhibitors. *Lancet* 1, 1405 (1962).
17. Dingle, H. R., Antihypertensive drugs and anaesthesia. *Anaesthesia* 21, 151 (1966).
18. Fieldman, E. J., Ridley, R. W. & Wood, E. H., Hemodynamic studies during thiopental sodium and nitrous oxide anesthesia in man. *Anesthesiology* 16, 473 (1955).
19. Prys-Roberts, C., Kelman, G. R. & Greenbaum R., The influence of circulatory factors on arterial oxygenation during anaesthesia in man. *Anaesthesia* 22, 257 (1967).
20. Etsten, B. & Li, T. H., Hemodynamic changes during thiopental in humans: cardiac

output, stroke volume, total peripheral resistance and intrathoracic blood volume. *J. clin. Invest.* 34, 500 (1955).

21. Prys-Roberts, C., Green, T. L., Meloche, R. & Foëx, P., Studies of anaesthesia in relation to hypertension. II: Haemodynamic consequences of induction and endotracheal intubation. *Brit. J. Anaesth.* 43, 6, 531, 1971.
22. Tomori, Z. & Widdicombe, J. G., Muscular, bronchomotor and cardiovascular reflexes elicited by mechanical stimulation of the respiratory tract. *J. Physiol. (Lond.)* 200, 25 (1969).
23. Corbett, J. L., Kerr, J. H. & Prys-Roberts, C., Cardiovascular responses to aspiration of secretions from the respiratory tract in man. *J. Physiol. (Lond.)* 201, 51 (1969).
24. Smith, A. C. & Spalding, J. M. K., Cardiovascular disturbances in severe tetanus due to overactivity of the sympathetic nervous system. *Anaesthesia* 24, 198 (1969).
25. Takeshima, K., Noda, K. & Higaki, M., Cardiovascular response to rapid anesthesia induction and endotracheal intubation, *Anesth. Analg. Curr. Res.* 43, 201 (1964).
26. Gersh, B. J., *Ventricular function and haemodynamica in the dog during anaesthesia.* (D. Phil. Thesis). Oxford 1970.
27. Gersh, B. J., Prys-Roberts, C., Reuben, S. R. & Baker, A. B., The relationship between depressed myocardial contractility and the stroke output of the canine heart during halothane anaesthesia, *Brit. J. Anaesth.* 42, 560 (1970).
28. Prys-Roberts, C., Gersh, B. J., Baker, A. B. & Reuben, S. R., Myocardial responses to direct and sympathetic nerve and receptor stimulation during halothane anaesthesia. *Brit. J. Anaesth.* 42, 560 (1970).
29. Wilcken, D. E. L., Charlier, A. A., Hoffman, J. I. E. & Guz, A., Effects of alterations in aortic impedance on the performance of the ventricles. *Circulat. Res.* 12, 283 (1964).

DRUG INTERACTIONS IN ANAESTHESIA

E. L. NOACH

Hardly any field of clinical medicine is as close to the pharmacologist as anaesthesiology. A majority of pharmacological studies are concerned with acute drug effects, for the obvious reason that test-objects such as isolated organs, do not survive for very long. The fact that the anaesthetist's main interest is also centered around acute drug effects often has little connection with his patients' survival, but nevertheless it gives him a similar approach to pharmacological aspects of his work. There are more points in common for both groups of workers, for instance their relationship to pharmacotherapy. Pharmacotherapy, in the strict sense of the word, means the elimination of disease in patients by drug treatment. It is only a remote consequence of the pharmacologist's effort: he provides others with the tools needed to achieve therapeutic success, and alas, in a pharmacologist's professional life the number of such successful tools created is only very small. The anaesthetist does not aim at pharmacotherapeutic success primarily, rather he provides one of the essential prerequisites within a wider therapeutic process. Of course in recent times the anaesthetist has become more and more involved in the fight against pain, so that nowadays he may be considered to be the expert in this domain of symptomatic pharmacotherapy, especially where other measures fail. However, he owes the ever-increasing demand on this skill to his experience of analgesic drug effects, collected in the course of his specialized approach to surgical patients.

Again a different use of drugs is made by the anaesthetist in preventing iatrogenic, pharmacogenic disease or disaster. When in the operating-theatre he administers drugs which prevent, say, ventricular fibrillation, he does not act as a substitute for the cardiologist who is not present, but rather as a pharmacologist eliminating the side effect of one drug by giving a different one.

Therefore, it is with good reasons that pharmacologists usually feel at home amongst anaesthetists. However, the pharmacologist may view the anaesthetist at work with mixed feelings: on the one hand he admires the skill and virtuosity with which the latter administers one drug after the other, often without the monitoring provided by the intricate experimental set-up of the pharmacological laboratory. On the other hand, if one considers the hazards of drug interactions encountered in animal experimentation, one tends, as a non-clinician, to consider the successful termination of any modern anaesthesia as a medical miracle. This feeling arises because pharmacologists are usually afraid of drug combinations, and in their analysis of the mechanism of drug action, they try to limit the number of variables to a minimum and preferably to one drug. They are aware of the possibility that the effect of a drug combination may outlast the usual duration of the effect of the components and they also know that often the effect of drug combinations is rather unpredictable.

It is within this context of a certain amount of insecurity that I will undertake to discuss different aspects of drug interactions in anaesthesia. Of course, the number of possible combinations is endless, and I will therefore limit this discussion to interactions of drugs commonly used in anaesthesia, with other drugs frequently encountered by the anaesthetist.

The effect of one drug on another drug's action is commonly referred to as synergism, antagonism, potentiation and so on. Although such a classification may be of practical value in the management of drugs already in use, it should be realized that this terminology is only descriptive and gives no explanation of the interaction. Hence, it does not provide a better understanding about the underlying processes. In a pharmacologist's opinion, it is important to have such an understanding in order to make a 'calculated guess' of interactions which might be expected to occur in combinations with new drugs. This lecture will therefore be mainly concerned with a classification based on the levels at which interactions take place, with examples taken from groups such as general anaesthesia, sedative drugs, analgesics and muscle relaxants.

LEVELS OF DRUG INTERACTION

In table 1, possible levels of drug interaction are summarized. *Category I,*

Table 1. Drug interactions

1. Chemical interaction
2. Interaction on level of drug receptors
3. Interaction due to drug-induced changes in physiological functions
4. Interaction due to drug-induced changes in absorption, distribution, metabolism or excretion of other drugs
5. Unknown mechanisms

direct chemical interaction, is perhaps the least important for the anaesthetist. In other fields, especially in toxicology, the effect of an active drug may be blocked by its precipitation – for instance the adstringent silver nitrate by sodium chloride – or by preventing its absorption. An example of the latter was recently found in our laboratory – the effect of folic acid on the antiepileptic drug diphenylhydantoin (phenytoin).

Category 2, interaction at the level of drug receptors, is more important. The principle is schematically shown in figure 1.

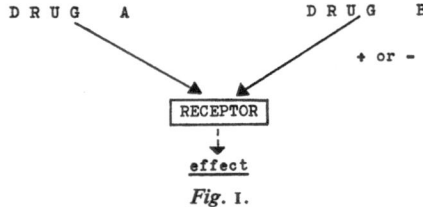

Fig. 1.

If two drugs ultimately act on the same receptor, some sort of modification of the effect of drug A by drug B has to be expected. This modification may be an enhancement, such as in figure 2, where the inherent blocking action

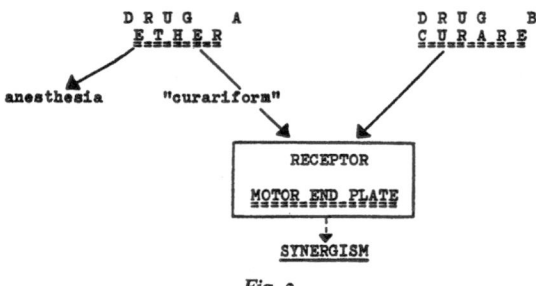

Fig. 2.

of ether on the motor end plate will help the neuromuscular blocking effect of curare. Hence less of the latter is required to provide muscular relaxation. Another example, which may be of practical importance, is that the antibiotics gentamycin and neomycin also have a neuromuscular blocking action (1) caused by a decrease in the release of acetylcholine from the nerve ending. This fact must be considered when patients receiving these antibiotics require surgery.

In figure 3 another example is given, showing that the general depression of the central nervous system by a neuroleptic drug such as chlorpromazine

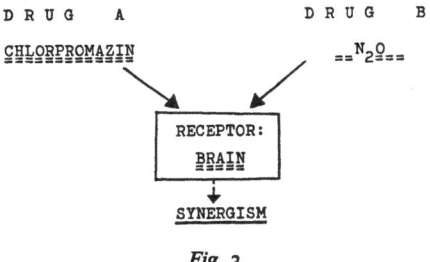

Fig. 3.

and also reserpine may enhance the anaesthetic effect of nitrous oxide (2). However, in this case, the nature of the receptor is less well understood than in the previous examples. In fact we do not know whether only one species of receptors is concerned, for instance in the cortex, or whether there are complementary effects on cortical neurones by nitrous oxide and receptors elsewhere, possibly in the brain stem, influenced by the neuroleptics.

A different example is shown in figure 4. Although here the interaction is

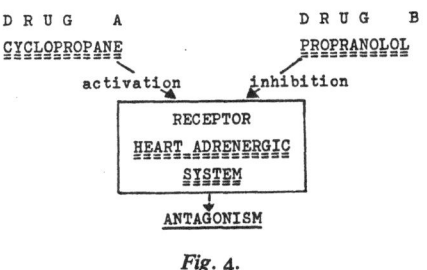

Fig. 4.

more complex than indicated in the schematic figure, we know that 'activation' by cyclopropane consists in sensitization of adrenergic receptors in the heart and elsewhere (3) to those actions of the sympathetic neurotransmitter which may precipitate cardiac fibrillation. This undesirable sympathetic effect may be prevented by the beta-blocker propranolol (4). This knowledge does not imply that all cardiac irregularities due to cyclopropane should be treated with propranolol; this depends on the anaesthetist's judgment, based on the knowledge of possible undesired side effects such as sudden bronchospasm in asthmatic patients.

The third category of drug interaction consists in alteration of the effects of the drug, by modifications of physiological functions elsewhere by other drugs. The general principle is illustrated in figure 5: the quantitative effect

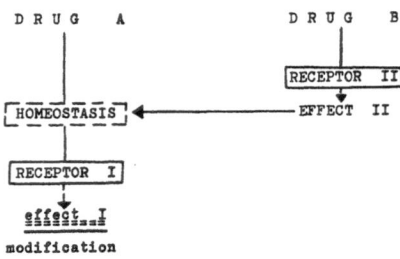

Fig. 5.

of a drug is always dependent on homeostatic mechanisms in the body, since such mechanisms determine the rate of delivery of the drug to its site of action. The transport of gaseous anaesthetics from the lungs to the brain is dependent on cardiovascular as well as pulmonary function. If, for example, gaseous exchange in the lungs is increased, more of the gaseous anaesthetic will be taken up in the blood. Amongst the group of drugs which may stimulate respiration, are the salicylates, especially if taken in high doses. In figure 6, the possible effects of hyperventilation are shown: more ether will be

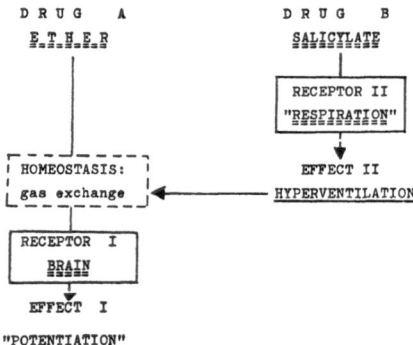

Fig. 6.

absorbed, and Bowman et al. (5) showed that salicylates 'potentiate' the effect of ether. That this is due to enhancement of respiratory uptake follows from the observation that injected anaesthetics, for instance pentobarbitone, are not potentiated by salicylates. It would be interesting to know whether this phenomenon, demonstrated in animal experiments, also occurs in clinical anaesthesia, for instance in patients treated with high doses of aspirin because of fever, pain or arthritis.

An interesting example in the same category – drug-induced modification of a homeostatic system which determines the effect of another drug – is concerned with cerebrospinal fluid flow. Drugs which act on the central nervous system may penetrate into the brain from the cerebrospinal fluid. If the fluid stream there is increased or decreased, there is less or more time, respectively, available for penetration. It is known that carbonic anhydrase inhibitors such as acetazolamide (Diamox) decrease the formation of cerebrospinal fluid. Since the total amount remains the same, this means that the flow of the liquid is slowed down, enabling drugs dissolved in it (having passed the choroid plexus) to get better access to the brain tissue. Reed (6) showed that during treatment with Diamox, the effect of pentobarbitone was prolonged proportionally with the decrease of liquor flow (Fig. 7). This

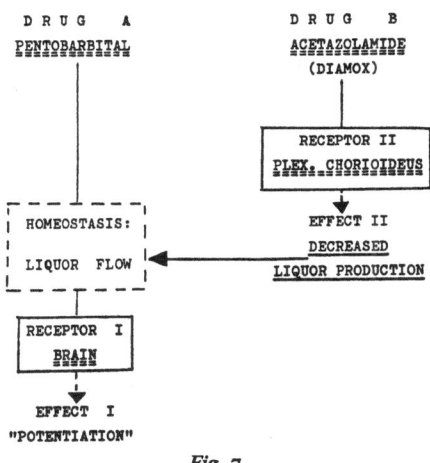

Fig. 7.

again was shown by animal experiments and it might be worth while to investigate whether patients regularly using oral diuretics require less of an anaesthetic.

The fourth category is the modification of the effect of one drug by changes in its absorption, distribution, metabolism and excretion, caused by another drug. This may be considered as one of the most important sources of interaction.

Absorption: Absorption from the gastro-intestinal tract can be decreased by several mechanisms. From medical school experiments you will remember that increased peristalsis brought about by laxatives, or adsorption of a drug by charcoal (norit), or putting a barrier of precipitated mucus on the intestinal epithelium by giving an adstringent, are all different ways to inhibit ab-

sorption. These mechanisms are mainly of interest in the treatment of intoxication and are of little importance in anaesthesiology. Drugs which improve
absorption have not properly been tried out. Recently it was discovered here
(7), that the anti-epileptic drug phenytoin (diphantoin) improves absorption
of substances such as NaCl and glucose. Experiments are being carried out
at present to see whether these findings may be extrapolated to other substances including drugs. It might be of value to remember this result, since if
the absorption of drugs such as barbiturates and analgesics is also enhanced,
one must be careful with the anaesthetic management of epileptic patients
on phenytoin.

Distribution: Modification of drug distribution is of great importance and
may be caused by several different mechanisms. One group of possibilities
has been mentioned already, namely, changes in homeostatic mechanisms
(examples: respiratory stimulation by salicylates and decreased cerebrospinal
fluid flow by acetazolamide). Marked changes in drug distribution may be
caused by interference with the *binding of a drug to blood proteins.* Many
drugs are transported in the blood whilst being loosely bound to serum proteins. This reversible binding has several consequences: it prevents the filtration of the drug by the glomeruli of the kidney, but also inhibits its rapid
penetration into the interstitial fluid. Therefore protein binding means that
there is a 'circulating depot' of the drug, protected against enzymatic breakdown. However, the protein binding is reversible and in the blood there is an
equilibrium between bound and free drug. Only the free fraction is biologi-
cally active, since it can traverse capillary walls, thus reaching the receptors,
and also the drug-metabolizing enzymes. Hence the amount of drug bound
to protein will gradually decrease. It should be remembered that the extent
of protein binding depends on certain physicochemical properties of the
drug, determining its affinity to the protein. If a second drug with a greater
affinity to the transport protein is administered, the first drug may be
'pushed away' from the protein. This means that the equilibrium:

protein-bound drug $\rightleftharpoons$ free drug

will be shifted to the right, thereby increasing the concentration of biologi-
cally active drug. This may be the basis of an effect caused by the administration of quinidine to animals recovering from the paralytic effects of curare.
Without an additional dose of curare, the animals suddenly become 're-
curarized' (8). Perhaps the same mechanism explains the enhancing effect of
the antidepressant imipramine (Tofranil) on barbiturate anaesthesia, although
other explanations have been proposed (9).

Shifting of the equilibrium between protein-bound and free drug may have effects which at first appear to be paradoxical. In table 2, the effect of the

Table 2. Effect of sulfinpyrazon (Enturen®) on plasma and brain concentrations of sulfa-ethyl-thiadiazol in the rat (derived from Anton (10).

Sulfinpyrazon		Sulfa-ethyl-thiadiazol	
Dose mg/kg	Plasma μg/ml	Plasma μg/ml	Brain μg/ml H_2O
0	0	194	5.1
25	140	143	5.6
50	270	120	7.9
100	500	80	8.8
200	700	75	9.2

anti-gout drug, sulfinpyrazon (Enturen) on blood and tissue levels of the chemotherapeutic sulfa-ethyl-thiadiazol is shown (10). Increasing doses of sulfinpyrazon will cause a parallel decrease in sulfa blood levels, whereas concentration of the sulfa in tissue increases: the drug is shifted from its protein-binding site and more free drug becomes available to diffuse out into the tissue.

From the examples given it may be evident that data on the degree of protein binding of a drug should be provided at the time of introduction of that drug. Unfortunately, in many cases our knowledge in this field is still quite deficient.

Metabolism: Having discussed changes in absorption and distribution, we now come to modifications of drug metabolism. In recent years, important discoveries have been made in this field. Axelrod (11) found that in the liver there is a special enzyme system which is mainly responsible for the oxidative breakdown of foreign substances. It is commonly called the 'liver microsomal drug metabolizing enzyme system' and many drugs are inactivated by it. The substances thus oxidized belong to nearly all classes of drugs. Some years later, the discovery was made that certain drugs enhance the disappearance of other drugs from the blood by activating this enzyme system (12, 13). This activation was found to be caused by the formation of enzyme molecules. Initially, only a few drugs were thought to be able to cause such an 'enzyme induction'; outstanding amongst these were phenobarbitone, and the carcinogenic agent 3.4.-benzpyrene. However, over the years, the list of substances with similar enzyme-inductory properties has grown considerably, and nowadays more than 200 such substances are

known. Not all of them are drugs; some are chemical substances in the environment which are able to stimulate liver enzymes, often causing their own
degradation in the body. Hepatic enzyme induction has to be looked upon
as a system of self-protection. It is fairly certain that people living in a
heavily polluted area such as Rijnmond, not only suffer from smog, but also
are better protected against systemic toxic effects than people living in
remote clean places.

Not all enzyme-inducing substances act in exactly the same way. However, it should be remembered that barbiturates are still amongst the most
powerful inducers. Even one administration of phenobarbitone may cause a
long-lasting increase in the liver's ability to break down many substances.
Among those is phenobarbitone itself and tolerance to many barbiturates is
at least partly due to this mechanism. Of the other drugs which are quickly
metabolized, anticoagulants of the coumarin group should be mentioned
(14, 15), see figure 8. This means that blood levels of coumarins will more

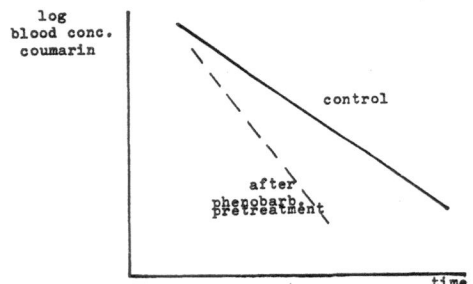

Fig. 8. Effect of hepatic enzyme induction by phenobarbital on elimination of coumarin
anticoagulants (schematic).

quickly decrease in patients treated with a barbiturate. Patients in hospital
frequently receive barbiturate hypnotics and this may mean that the dose of
anticoagulant may need to be elevated in order to get the appropriate blood
level. Once they have left the hospital and are sleeping better at home, the
barbiturate can be stopped and its effect on liver enzymes gradually wears off.
If these patients are not regularly controlled by a thrombosis service, they may
get symptoms of coumarin overdosage. Therefore, during the pre-operative
management of patients, one should consider the effects of enzyme-inducing
drugs on agents used in anaesthesia. It has been shown for instance that the
metabolic dechlorination of halothane is increased after the use of pentobarbitone (16). Since under normal conditions in man, about 20% of the administered dose of halothane is broken down in the body (17), increase of

metabolic conversion may mean that more has to be administered to patients regularly using phenobarbitone.

Apart from the drugs which cause an increase in drug metabolism, we know others which are able to inhibit the metabolic inactivation of other drugs. The best known among those is a compound usually indicated as SKF 525–A (beta-diethylaminoethyl– 2.2.diphenylpentanoate). Since no practical use is made of such an inhibition, this will not be discussed further.

Excretion: The last mechanism of interaction to be discussed is modification in the excretion of drugs. A well-known example is the inhibition of renal excretion of penicillin by probenecid. Since nowadays there is no lack of penicillin, this inhibition is rarely used.

Much less is known about the fact that the excretion of drugs by the kidneys can be altered by changing the pH of the urine. As an example, barbital (Veronal, diethyl barbituric acid) is a weak acid, which in an acid medium is hardly ionized, but in an alkaline medium most of it is dissociated. It is known that barbital is excreted in its unchanged form, being filtered by the glomeruli and varying amounts being reabsorbed in the renal tubules. The degree of reabsorption depends on the pH in the tubular lumen. In order to understand this, it should be said that in this case reabsorption is a passive diffusion through the cell membrane. This will happen only if the substance is sufficiently lipoid-soluble, since the cell membrane contains lipids. Because the unionized moiety is more lipophilic than the barbiturate anion, little will be reabsorbed if the urine is alkaline, see figure 9. In al-

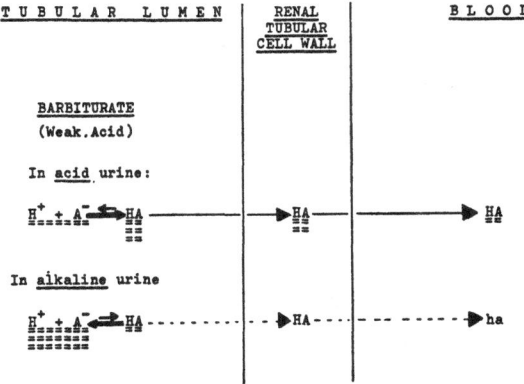

Fig. 9. Influence of urinary pH on renal excretion of weak electrolyte.

kaline urine most of the barbiturate will be dissociated, but in an acid urine the barbiturate will be unionized and will readily diffuse back into the blood. It is clear that this process, analysed by Brodie and his co-workers (18, 19), can easily be applied in the clinic. By the very simple method of administering NH_4Cl to acidify, or $NaHCO_3$ to alkalinise the urine, we may profoundly alter the excretion of drugs. This is especially of value in the treatment of intoxication by barbiturates or other ionizable drugs. Now that this mechanism has become more generally known, information about the degree of dissociation of drugs at body pH may be obtained from most drug manufacturers. Application of the principle mentioned may be life-saving.

The field of drug interactions is without limits, even if we only consider those interactions which may occur in clinical practice. In our 'drug-taking' society, many people consider that taking sleeping-pills, tranquillizers, energisers, etc. is part of their normal menu and will not even mention it when questioned by the doctor about the use of drugs. This omission may occasionally cause unexpected effects of drugs administered by the physician.

Few people have such a good memory that they will remember all possible interaction effects. It has been the purpose of this lecture to discuss broad categories of interaction, which will be of value to anaesthetists. We as pharmacologists like to say that there is no special pharmacological technique in existence, but we borrow everything in methodology from physiology, biochemistry, behavioural sciences and so on. The only specificity of pharmacology is a peculiar way of thinking about drugs. I hope that my lecture has been a contribution to your ability to think pharmacologically so that it will help our mutual co-operation and understanding.

REFERENCES

1. Brazil, O. V. & Prado, F. J., *Arch. Int. Pharmacodyn.* 179, 65 (1969).
2. Rummel, W. & Wellensiek, H. J., *Arch. Int. Pharmacodyn.* 122, 339 (1959).
3. Gravenstein, J. S., Sherman, E. T. & Andersen, T. W., *J. Pharmacol. exp. Ther.* 129, 428 (1960).
4. Lewis, G. B. H., *Canad. Anesth. Soc. J.* 16, 547 (1969).
5. Bowman, D. C., Damgaard, E. D. & Doemling, D. B., *J. Pharmacol. exp. Ther.* 138, 236 (1962).
6. Reed, D. J., *Arch. Int. Pharmacodyn.* 171, 206 (1968).
7. Plevier, W., van Rees, H., de Wolff, F. A. & Noach, E. L., unpublished observations.
8. Schmidt, J. L., Vick, N. A. & Sadove, M. S., *J. Amer. med. Ass.* 183, 669, (1963).
9. Kato, R., Chiesara, E. & Vassanelli, P., *Bioch. Pharmacol.* 12, 357 (1963).
10. Anton, A. H., *J. Pharmacol. exp. Ther.* 134, 291 (1961).
11. Axelrod, J., *J. biol. Chem.* 214, 753 (1955).
12. Remmer, H., *Naunyn-Schmiedebergs Arch. exp. Path. Pharmak.* 235, 279 (1959).

13. Conney, A. H. & Burns, J. J., *Advances in Pharmacol.* 1, 31 (1962).
14. MacDonald, M. G. & Robinson, D. S., *J. Amer. med. Ass.* 204, 97 (1968).
15. Weiner, M., *Nature (London)* 212, 1599 (1966).
16. Van Dyke, R. A., *J. Pharmacol. exp. Ther.* 154, 364 (1966).
17. Rehder, K., Forbes, J., Alter, H., Hessler, O. & Stier, A., *Anesthesiology* 28, 711 (1967).
18. Brodie, B. B. & Hogben, C. A. M., *J. Pharm. Pharmacol.* 9, 345 (1957).
19. Schanker, L. S., *Pharmacol. Rev.* 14, 501 (1962).

ON THE TOXICITY OF HALOTHANE

B. R. SIMPSON, L. STRUNIN AND B. WALTON

The history of anaesthesia contains many instances of strongly held beliefs which have subsequently not been substantiated. For example, many children died during anaesthesia because the particular difficulties associated with this age group were not appreciated and death was attributed to a condition named 'status lymphaticus' (1); it is clear now that no such condition exists. Similarly for many years it was argued that spinal anaesthesia led to irreversible damage to nerve tissue; this is now known to be avoidable (2). Also it was alleged that the administration of a general anaesthetic to an elderly person frequently led to irreversible central nervous system damage; this has now been refuted (3).

It is of interest therefore that a cause and effect relationship between the administration of halothane and post-operative liver damage has been claimed. However, much of the evidence which has been presented in favour of this relationship does not withstand careful scrutiny and it is the aim of this paper to review the arguments for and against 'halothane hepatitis' as a specific entity.

Table 1. causes of post-operative hepatic morbidity

1. Pre-existing factors	Liver disease, heart failure, malnutrition, drug therapy
2. Premedication	Narcotics, diuretics, blood transfusion
3. Anaesthesia	Physiological changes, hypotension, hypoxia, blood loss and vasopressors, anaesthetic agents
4. Operation	Site of operation, surgical mishap
5. Post-operative factors	Anoxaemia and acid base balance, narcotics, antibiotics, diuretics, steroids and blood transfusion

Many factors may be involved (Table 1) when a patient develops jaundice following anaesthesia and surgery, and all anaesthetic agents and techniques in common use have been incriminated (Table 2). Furthermore, Henderson and Gordon (4) have shown that the incidence of post-operative liver damage has risen in the last two decades (Table 3). This increase, which has occurred

Table 2. Liver damage following anaesthesia.

Agent	Author	Year
Cyclopropane	Bennike et al.	1964
Diethyl ether	Dawson et al.	1963
Divinyl ether	Hawk et al.	1941
Epidural	Gingrich and virtue	1964
Local	Caravati and Wotton	1962
Methoxyflurane	Lindenbaum and Liefer	1963
Spinal	Keeri-szanto and Lafleur	1963
Thiopentone, nitrous oxide, suxamethonium	Herber and Specht	1965
Tribromethanol	Andersen	1945
Trichlorethylene	Herdman	1945

Table 3. Incidence of post-operative jaundice.

	Jaundice per 1000
1953–1956	1.1
1960–1963	4.2

1960–1963	Jaundice per 1000
Halothane	4.1
$N_2O \pm$ relaxant	4.1
Cyclopropane	7.4

regardless of the anaesthetic agents used, has been attributed to the increasing complexity of surgical operations and the wider use of blood transfusion and potentially hepatotoxic drugs other than anaesthetic agents. Nevertheless, since halothane was first introduced in 1956 (5) a steady trickle of clinical reports has appeared alleging a cause and effect relationship between halothane and post-operative liver damage. These reports led to a number of retrospective surveys, the largest of which was the United States National Halothane Study (6).

This study (6) reviewed the incidence of fatal massive hepatic necrosis occurring within six weeks of anaesthesia in some 850,000 patients undergoing surgery in 34 hospitals. About 250,000 of these patients received halothane. Eighty-two cases of fatal massive hepatic necrosis were recorded of which all but nine could be explained on the basis of either the patient's known disease or the surgical procedure or a recognizable post-operative complication. Hence nine cases were attributed to the anaesthetic agent; seven of these nine unexplained cases had received halothane and four of the seven had previously received halothane within six weeks of the final operative procedure. Reports on four of these seven cases, however, had already been published, and two others were known to the participating hospitals before the start of the study. So from this extensive review only one new case of massive hepatic necrosis associated with halothane was elicited. The committee concluded that 'unexplained fever and jaundice in a specific patient might reasonably be considered a contra-indication to its subsequent use'. Later Dykes and Bunker (7) drew attention to the fact that 'there was not a single patient in the National Halothane Study who was jaundiced after the administration of halothane, who died after a second administration, and who was found at necropsy to have suffered massive or intermediate hepatic necrosis'.

A statistic from this study concerning the incidence of fatal massive hepatic necrosis attributed to halothane is widely quoted. The overall incidence of massive hepatic necrosis was approximately 1 in 10,000 – that is 82 in 850,000 – regardless of the anaesthetic agent used; but in only nine of these patients – of whom seven received halothane – was it felt that massive hepatic necrosis could be attributed to the anaesthetic agent itself. Therefore at worst the true incidence of massive hepatic necrosis associated with halothane in this series was seven out of 250,000 or about 1 in 35,000, and not, as is sometimes stated, 1 in 10,000. It must also be recognized that the knowledge of the "pre-existence" of six of these seven cases may have prejudiced the validity of this statistic.

Halothane is now administered in 70-90% of all anaesthetics in those countries where it is freely available (8). Since liver damage after surgery and anaesthesia is increasing it is not surprising that in spite of the reassurance of the early reviews and clinical reports, further studies, reviews and leading articles have attempted to link the administration of halothane – particularly multiple – with liver dysfunction. It is difficult to place the data from some of these studies in perspective – for example Trey and his colleagues (9, 10) did not relate the number of patients who died with massive hepatic necrosis to the total number of patients who received halothane. Several of the surveys depend on second-hand information and the risk inherent in relying on such reports in exemplified by a recent paper entitled 'Hepatic Necrosis Associated with Halothane Anesthesia' (11); persual of the case histories in this paper reveals that two of eight patients quoted did not in fact receive halothane.

A small series of patients subjected to multiple halothane anaesthetics for radium treatment of carcinoma of the cervix uteri was reviewed by Hughes and Powell (12). They described a greater than 2% incidence of severe liver damage. However, if this high incidence in fact had been related to the administration of halothane, one would have expected similar findings from other centres, since up to the present time halothane has been a part of more than 50 million anaesthetics.

Sharpstone and his colleagues (13) reported recently a series of 11 cases of post-operative jaundice in which nine patients had unexplained fever, and three had jaundice after previous halothane administration. All the patients became jaundiced after further administration of halothane, and six died of massive hepatic necrosis. Halothane was thought to be responsible, although five of the patients had a malignant disease, one had cholelithiasis with a subphrenic abscess and one had cirrhosis of the liver. Hill (14) subsequently pointed out that this latter patient had developed a severe urinary infection after his first halothane anaesthetic and thus his post-operative fever was hardly unexplained.

The view that unexplained post-operative fever after halothane should preclude its subsequent administration is supported by Sharpstone et al. (13). However, Trey and his colleagues (9) showed that post-operative fever is as common after other anaesthetic agents as it is after halothane and this was confirmed by Dykes (15) who described a variety of post-operative raised temperature patterns regardless of the agent used. Furthermore, a retrospective survey (16) has described eight patients who became jaundiced after halothane, in four of whom subsequent exposure did not lead to a recurrence of the jaundice.

A recent review by Sherlock (17) concluded that 'halothane hepatitis' may be differentiated from viral hepatitis on clinical, morbid anatomical and immunological grounds. However, the arguments put forward are not convincing. The author's clinical criteria include the occurrence of unexplained post-operative fever, an association with multiple exposure to halothane, a number of nonspecific changes in liver function and jaundice which may or may not be present. The lack of specificity and significance of post-operative fever has already been mentioned, and the morbid anatomical differences seem to depend for recognition on 'the experience of the pathologist'. The immunological differentiation is based on the association of anti-mitochondrial antibodies and induced lymphocyte transformation with 'halothane hepatitis'. These tests are, however, non-specific, and furthermore the suggestion that a negative test for hepatitis-association antigen (Australia antigen, HAA) rules out coincidental viral hepatitis is not supported by other expert opinion (18, 19).

Reports of bronchospasm, skin rashes, arthralgia, unexplained fever, leukocytosis and eosinophilia in association with post-halothane jaundice, were mentioned by Doniach (20) as evidence for the hypothesis that a hypersensitivity to halothane may be involved in such cases. Bronchospasm is a term often used loosely to describe airway obstruction from many causes. Arthralgia, fever, skin rashes and leukocytosis have also been described in association with viral hepatitis (21) and therefore their occasional appearance following anaesthesia does not help to distinguish viral infection from hypersensitivity as a cause of post-operative jaundice. Although a systematic search for eosinophilia was recommended, it is of interest that Sharpstone and his colleagues (13) found no evidence of eosinophilia among their eleven cases.

The Committee on Safety of Drugs collects reports of adverse reactions to drugs occurring in Great Britain, and since 1964, 126 cases of jaundice associated with anaesthesia have been reported. Of these only 103 relate to halothane (22), although Mushin and his colleagues (8) stated, that in Great Britain, halothane now forms a part in nearly 90% of all general anaesthetics. These authors recently reported a statistical comparison between three groups of patients – a control group of surgical patients, 54 patients reported to the Committee on Safety of Drugs during the period 1964-1969 and 74 patients from the literature. The latter two groups were patients who had become jaundiced after multiple halothane anaesthetics and, within these groups there was an apparent excess of patients who had had two anaesthetics within one month. They concluded that 'halothane should, if possible be avoided in patients who have had it before, particularly if this was within the previous four weeks'.

This study was based on the hypothesis that 'halothane hepatitis' is a sensitisation phenomenon and therefore no clinical details of the patients were provided. It is important to note that all cases of jaundice associated with halothane reported to the Committee on Safety of Drugs were included. The crux of the matter is, however, whether or not the jaundice in these cases was unexplained. The National Halothane Study (6) reported 82 cases of fatal post-operative massive hepatic necrosis, but in only nine of these did the expert panel decide that no alternative adequate explanation existed other than the anaesthesia. These data suggest that only some 10% of post-operative liver damage is likely to be attributable to the anaesthetic agent. Similarly, we are currently engaged in a study of post-operative jaundice occurring in Great Britain and Eire, and to date in most cases investigated, the jaundice may well be due to factors other than the anaesthetic agent. It is unlikely, therefore, that all the cases reported to the Committee on Safety of Drugs were in fact unexplained and the apparent excess figure of 68% (8) of the total cases of jaundice reported to the Committee or who became jaundiced after two operations within a month – with an alleged cause and effect relationship with halothane – should be considerably reduced. In addition, the two groups of patients reported to the Committee and collected from the literature were limited to anaesthetics repeated within 10 years, and it is therefore misleading to include in the calculations the 23% of the control group who received their penultimate anaesthetic more than ten years previously. Recalculation shows that 13% of the control group, and not the 7% stated (8), received 2 anaesthetics within one month. Thus the apparent excess of patients who became jaundiced after two operations within a month, with an alleged cause and effect relationship with halothane may not exist. However, the high incidence of jaundice after operations repeated within a month remains a matter of concern. It is of interest therefore that a finding from the National Halothane Study (6) demonstrates that repeated low risk operations have an unexpectedly high mortality, regardless of the anaesthetic agents used (Table 4).

Table 4. Crude overall post-operative death rates per 10,000.

Operation	No previous general anaesthesia	Previous non-halothane	Previous halothane
Low-death-rate	18	82	84
Mid-death-rate	193	461	431
High-death-rate	868	1354	1183

In contrast, an early study by Mushin and his colleagues (23), and more recent ones by Dykes (16) and Gronert (24) and others could not demonstrate an association between multiple halothane anaesthetics and liver damage. Furthermore, cases have been reported where post-operative liver dysfunction might have been attributed to halothane, had not other aetiological factors subsequently come to light (25, 26). Finally, it must be remembered that, as Dykes and Walzer (27) pointed out, a small percentage of patients can be expected to be suffering coincidentally from hepatic dysfunction not suspected pre-operatively, but revealing itself during the post-operative period.

PRESENT POSITION

Halothane is used in over 70% of all anaesthetic procedures in countries where it is freely available. Thus, one might expect halothane to have been administered in most cases where post-operative liver damage occurs. The United States National Halothane Study (6) showed that the great majority of cases of massive hepatic necrosis were attributable to causes other than the anaesthetic agent used. Nevertheless there remains a small number of cases for whom no adequate explanation exists. Two groups of patients give cause for concern. Firstly, overweight, middle aged patients with a vague history of indigestion, and secondly patients submitted to multiple halothane anaesthetics, often for minor surgical procedures.

If halothane and liver damage are related, at least four possible mechanisms must be considered: a direct toxic effect; a normal or abnormal metabolite; a relation to viral hepatitis; and hypersensitivity either to halothane itself or to a normal or abnormal metabolite thereof.

DIRECT TOXIC EFFECT

A direct hepatotoxin should fulfill criteria which include the following conditions (28):

a. Liver damage of a distinct histological pattern appearing after a predictable and usually brief latent period following exposure to the offending agent.
b. The damage is elicited in all exposed individuals and can be reproduced in experimental animals.
c. Damage is dose related and other tissues are often affected.

Halothane fulfills none of these conditions, and large quantities have been ingested by man without ill effect (29, 30).

NORMAL OR ABNORMAL METABOLITE

Halothane is metabolised by man (31, 32) and other species, and a metabolite could act as a hepatotoxin either in the form of a free radical or as a cumulative toxic substance. A metabolite could also act as a hapten and thus lead to a hypersensitivity response (See below).

If the causal agent were a normal metabolite, the criteria laid down for a hepatotoxin should be fulfilled. Furthermore, if an abnormal metabolite was involved, one would expect a familial or genetic association to have been demonstrated; this had not been the case. By way of contrast in malignant hyperpyrexia, which may be triggered by halothane, although only about

170 cases have been reported in the literature (33), genetic and familial links have already been clearly established.

None of the known metabolites of halothane has been shown to be hepatotoxic in animals (34). Enzyme induction (35) and genetic and environmental factors (36) have been shown to influence the normal rate of halothane metabolism in man, but no evidence has been published to suggest that these factors are associated with liver damage.

RELATION TO VIRAL HEPATITIS

The incidence of viral hepatitis (infectious and serum) in the world is unknown. The disease appears to be becoming more prevalent, and Harville and Summerskill (37) reported that 80% of their patients were over 40. This age group is the one particularly associated with the halothane dilemma.

The discovery of the hepatitis-associated antigen (Australia antigen, HAA) initially led to the expectation that a satisfactory diagnostic test for viral hepatitis had been found (38). However, it is now becoming clear that hepatitis associated antigen is probably only associated with serum (or long-incubation) hepatitis (38), and furthermore, as the test is not technically straightforward the percentage of positive results varies widely from laboratory to laboratory. The antigen may only be found transiently, even in confirmed cases. Jaundice may also be associated with viruses other than those responsible for infectious and serum hepatitis, for example cytomegalovirus (39) – for which again there is no satisfactory test. It is clear, therefore that a negative test for hepatitis associated antigen does not appear to rule out viral infection.

Dykes and Bunker (7) estimate that in the United States of America 200-300 patients are likely to be subjected to anaesthesia while incubating viral hepatitis, and the potential effect of anaesthesia on such patients, or on those with chronic active hepatitis, is not clear. It has also been estimated that one patient in 30,000 anaesthetised may coincidentally develop viral hepatitis during the month following anaesthesia (40). Furthermore published evidence indicates that the ratio of sub-clinical to overt cases may be 12:1 (41) and that, in the healthy population, the carrier rate may be greater than 6% (42). In the light of this evidence the hypothesis that all cases of 'halothane hepatitis' are in fact viral in origin (43) is not unreasonable. It has also been suggested that carriers of viral infection, while normally being symptom free, may manifest clinical signs post-operatively owing to non-specific depression of their normal immunological responses by surgery and anaesthesia (44). Is it possible that halothane depresses immunological responses more than other agents?

It has recently been claimed (45, 46, 47) that liver damage due to viral infection can be differentiated from that caused by halothane either on clinico-pathological or morbid anatomical grounds alone. Unfortunately, in all studies, the pathologists were in possession of all the clinical and biochemical details before studying the liver sections by light and electron microscopy. In contrast, where the liver sections were unlabelled and clinical histories were not available, the expert pathologists associated with the National Halothane Study were unable to distinguish between massive hepatic necrosis occurring after viral hepatitis and that alleged to occur after halothane anaesthesia (48).

Until liver damage in patients with alleged halothane hepatitis can be clearly distinguished from that seen in viral hepatitis, or unequivocal diagnostic tests are devised for the possible viruses involved, it remains impossible to positively exclude a viral aetiology in any individual case.

HYPERSENSITIVITY

If a drug acts as an antigen in initiating a hypersensitivity response, certain criteria should be satisfied:

a. The drug should be a large or a highly reactive small molecule, this latter being capable of combining with proteins or other molecules in the body, or be metabolised to a substance which can do the same.
b. Rashes, eosinophilia, arthralgia, fever and other signs of hypersensitivity should be commonly seen.
c. There is usually a history of previous exposure to the antigen.
d. Hypersensitivity, once established, is usually long-standing, although delayed hypersensitivity tends to diminish with time.

Halothane is a small, chemically unreactive, poorly water-soluble molecule. Neither halothane itself, nor any metabolite thereof has been shown to combine with proteins or other large molecules. It has been suggested that halothane combines with mitochondria (49), but recent work by Schumer and his colleagues (50) demonstrates that halothane does not induce any long-lasting impairment of liver mitochondrial function. The various criteria of hypersensitivity have been neither consistently nor commonly observed. The difficulty in interpreting rashes, fever and eosinophilia associated with surgery and anaesthesia, has already been mentioned. Hypersensitivity responses usually occur after multiple exposures, although such responses may occur after a single exposure – for example after chlorpromazine. However, chlorpromazine combines with mitochondria (51) – and could thus act as a hapten, and furthermore, genetic links have been demonstrated (52). Once drug hypersensitivity is established, further exposure leads to a reaction in a high percentage of cases – for instance 40% with chlorpromazine (52). Dykes and his colleagues (16) reported four patients, in all of whom, although liver dysfunction followed an initial exposure to halothane, subsequent re-exposure did not lead to further damage. It has been suggested (53) that 'halothane hypersensitivity' persists for only 2-3 months, and the interval between anaesthetics was longer than this in two of these four patients. Burns (54) also recently reported two patients who became jaundiced after their second halothane anaesthetic, but not after their third exposure.

Tests alleging the presence of an immunological response to halothane include anti-mitochondrial antibodies in relatively high titre, and induced lymphocyte transformation. The tests for antimitochondrial antibodies have been positive in only some of the cases of alleged 'halothane hepatitis' (49, 55, 56) and antimitochondrial antibodies may be found in a variety of other liver disorders (49, 56). The fact that carbon-tetrachloride administration to rats produces anti-mitochondrial antibodies (56) suggests that these antibodies may be a nonspecific result of liver damage. The implication is that liver damage releases tissue-specific antigen to which the subjects may not have acquired a full immunological tolerance.

Lymphocyte stimulation by specific antigens in clinical hypersensitivity and by plant mitogens may result in increased uptake of tritiated thymidine by cultured cells. Paronetto and Popper (55) used this test to study 15 patients with alleged 'halothane hepatitis' and showed lymphocyte stimulation in ten and inhibition in three others. Some of the positive levels of stimulation were only marginally higher than the upper limit of their normal controls and the highest levels were recorded in two patients after single exposure – one to halothane and one to methoxyflurane. The implications of these findings is that halothane itself is the antigen, since it was used to provoke the lymphocyte stimulation in these patients. It is of interest to note that the period of stimulation was short and confined to the period of jaundice. This raises the question as to whether lymphocyte stimulation may be nonspecific to some types of liver disease, rather than indicative of the cause. Park and his colleagues (43) recently showed that surgery provokes a biphasic response in lymphocyte stimulation. For the first few days post-operatively the level of stimulation is depressed, but subsequently the lymphocytes show a degree of stimulation far higher than the pre-operative level. It is possible that Paronetto and Popper (55) were merely demonstrating this 'normal' rise in lymphocyte responsiveness after surgery and the liver dysfunction in their patients was coincidental.

Halothane hypersensitivity has been alleged to have developed in a few anaesthetists, other operating room personnel and one worker manufacturing halothane. One case was reported in detail (57), in which an initial illness diagnosed as viral hepatitis was followed by recurrent attacks of hepatitis allegedly due to halothane, culminating in a further attack following a challenge with the agent. The case history reveals, however, that although this person frequently relapsed soon after re-exposure on at least one occasion he was exposed to halothane for some time without ill effect. A possible alternative diagnosis in this case is chronic active hepatitis and it is unfortunate, therefore, that tests for smooth muscle antibody (58) and hepatitis associated antigen were not reported subsequently. It must also be noted that this person was not challenged with agents other than halothane.

The evidence against hypersensitivity in operating room personnel must also be born in mind. Halothane is present in the atmosphere of well-ventilated North American operating rooms (59) and has been detected in the blood (60) and expired air (59, 60) of operating room personnel and metabolites have been found in their urine (59). However, a survey (61) of the causes of death of 441 American anaesthesiologists presented no evidence of a higher incidence of liver disorders in this group when compared with a general population sample. In view of the large number of operating room personnel exposed to halothane, it is surprising that so few alleged reactions have been reported.

CONCLUSION

The scientific evidence for the existence of 'halothane hepatitis' is incomplete. If it does exist, it is rare. Viral hepatitis cannot at present be ruled out in any individual case. It would seem reasonable to expect that halothane, like all other anaesthetic agents, must carry some small risk of causing post-operative liver dysfunction.

Further detailed accurate information is needed about all cases of liver dysfunction occurring after any anaesthetic procedure to enable the extent of the problem to be determined and its mechanism to be elucidated.

Meanwhile, the charge against halothane remains, as in Scottish law – not proven.

REFERENCES

1. Adriani, J., In: *The pharmacology of anesthetic drugs*. p. 126. Springfield (Ill.) 1952.
2. Dripps, R. D. & Vandam, L. D., Long term follow-up of patients who received 10,098 spinal anaesthetics; failure to discover major neurological sequelae. *J. Amer. med. Ass.* 156, 1486 (1954).
3. Simpson, B. R., Williams, M., Scott, J. F. & Crampton-Smith, A., *Lancet* 2, 887 (1961).
4. Henderson, J. C. & Gordon, R. A., The incidence of post-operative jaundice with special reference to halothane. *Can. Anaesth. Soc. J.* 11, 453 (1964).
5. Raventos, J., The action of fluothane – a new volatile anaesthetic. *Brit. J. Pharmacol.* 11, 394 (1956).
6. Subcommittee of the National Academy of Sciences. *J. Amer. med. Ass.* 197, 775 (1966).
7. Dykes, M. H. M. & Bunker, J. P., Hepatotoxicity and anaesthetics. *Pharmacol. Physicians* 4, 1 (1970).
8. Mushin, W. W., Rosen, M. & Jones, E. V., Post-halothane jaundice in relation to previous administration of halothane. *Brit. med. J.* 1, 18 (1971).
9. Trey, C., Lipworth, L., Chalmers, T. C., Davidson, C. S., Gotlieb, L. S., Popper, H. & Saunders, S. J., Fulminant hepatic failure – presumably contribution of halothane. *New Eng. J. Med.*, 279, 798 (1968).
10. Trey, C. & Davidson, C. S., Co-operative study of fulminant hepatitis. *Clin. Res.* 2, 462 (1969).
11. Peters, R. L., Edmonson, H. A., Reynolds, T. B., Meister, J. C. and Curphey, T. J., Hepatic necrosis associated with halothane anesthesia. *Amer. J. Med.*, 47, 748 (1969).
12. Hughes, M. & Powell, L. W., Recurrent hepatitis in patients receiving multiple halothane anaesthetics for radium treatment of carcinoma of the cervix uteri. *Gastroenterology* 58, 790 (1970).
13. Sharpstone, P., Medley, D. R. K. & Williams, R., Halothane hepatitis – a preventable disease? *Brit. med. J.* 1, 448 (1971).
14. Hill, J. D., Halothane hepatitis. *Brit. med. J.* 2, 166 (1971).
15. Dykes, M. H. M., Unexplained post-operative fever – its value as a sign of halothane sensitization. *J. Amer. med. Ass.* 216, 641 (1971).
16. Dykes, M. H. M., Walzer, S. G., Slater, E. M., Gibson, J. M. & Ellis, D. S., Acute parenchymatous hepatic disease following general anaesthesia. *J. Amer. med. Ass.* 193, 339 (1965).
17. Sherlock, S., Progress report halothane hepatitis. *Gut* 12, 324 (1971).
18. Shulman, N. R., Hepatitis associated antigen. *Amer. J. Med.* 49, 669 (1970).
19. Wright, R., The Australia (hepatitis) antigen. *Brit. J. Hosp. Med.* 4, 75 (1970).
20. Doniach, D., Cell-mediated immunity in halothane hypersensitivity. *New Eng. J. Med.* 283, 315 (1970).
21. Mosley, J. W. & Galambos, J. T. In: *Diseases of the liver*. pp. 448, 451, 453. Philadelphia (Pa) 1959.
22. Inman, W. H. W., personal communication (1971).
23. Mushin, W. W., Rosen, M., Bowen, D. J. & Campbell, H., Halothane and liver dysfunction. A retrospective survey. *Brit. med. J.* 2, 329 (1964).
24. Gronert, G. A., Schaner, P. J. & Gunther, R. C., Multiple halothane anaesthesia in the burn patient. *J. Amer. med. Ass.* 205, 878 (1968).
25. Hege, M. J. D., Halothane anaesthesia in a patient with acute hepatic disease. *Anesthesiology* 32, 170 (1970).

26. Marx, G. F., Nagayoshi, M., Shoukas, J. A. & Wollman, S. B., Unsuspected infectious hepatitis in surgical patients. *J. Amer. med. Ass.* 205, 169 (1968).

27. Dykes, M. H. M. & Walzer, S. G., Pre-operative and post-operative hepatic dysfunction. *Surg. Gynec. Obstet.* 124, 747 (1967).

28. Klatskin, G., Toxic and drug induced hepatitis. In: *Diseases of the Liver*, 3rd edition, Philadelphia (Pa) & Toronto 1969.

29. Kopriva, C. J. & Lowenstein, E., An anaesthetic accident: cardiovascular collapse from liquid halothane delivery. *Anesthesiology* 30, 246-247 (1969).

30. Curelani, I., Stanciu, S. T., Nicolau, V., Fuhrer, H. & Iliescu, M., A case of recovery from coma produced by ingestion of 250 ml of halothane. *Brit. J. Anaesth.* 40, 283 (1968).

31. Van Dyke, R. A., Chenoweth, M. B. & Van Poznak, A., Metabolism of volatile anesthetics – I. *Biochem. Pharmacol.* 13, 1239 (1964).

32. Rehder, K., Forbes, J., Alter, H., Hessler, O. & Stier, A., Halothane biotransformation in man: a quantitative study. *Anesthesiology* 28, 711 (1967).

33. Britt, B. A. & Kalow, W., Malignant hyperthermia: a statistical review. *Canad. Anaesth. Soc. J.* 17, 293 (1970).

34. Airaksinen, M. M. & Tammisto, T., Toxic actions of the metabolites of halothane: LD_{50} and some metabolic effects of trifluoroethanol and trifluoroacetic acid in mice and guinea pigs. *Ann. Med. exp. Fenn.* 46, 242 (1968).

35. Cascorbi, H. F., Blake, D. A. & Helrich, M., Differences in the biotransformation of halothane in man. *Anesthesiology* 32, 119 (1970).

36. Cascorbi, H. F., Vesell, E. S., Blake, D. A. & Helrich, M., Genetic and environmental influence on halothane metabolism in twins. *Clin. Pharm. Therapeut.* 12, 50 (1970).

37. Harville, D. D. & Summerskill, W. H. J., Surgery in acute hepatitis: Causes and effects. *J. Amer. med. Ass.* 184, 257 (1963).

38. Blumberg, B. S., Sutnick, A. I., Londin, W. T. & Millman, I., Australia antigen and hepatitis. *New Eng. J. Med.* 283, 349 (1970).

39. Kantor, G. L. & Johnson, B. L., Cytomegalovirus infection associated with cardiopulmonary bypass. *Arch. Int. Med.* 125, 488 (1970).

40. Bunker, J. P. & Blumenfeld, C. M., Liver necrosis after halothane (Fluothane) anaesthesia. Cause or Coincidence? *New Eng. J. Med.* 268, 531 (1963).

41. Eisenstein, A. B., Aach, R. A., Jacobsohn, W. & Goldman, A., Infectious hepatitis in a general hospital. *J. Amer. med. Ass.* 185, 171 (1963).

42. Capps, R. B., Sborov, V. & Scheiffley, C. S., A syringe transmitted epidemic of infectious hepatitis. *J. Amer. med. Ass.* 136, 819 (1948).

43. Vickers, M. D. & Dinnick, O. P., Post-operative hepatic morbidity with special reference to the role of halothane. *Anaesthesia* 20, 29 (1966).

44. Park, S. K., Wallace, H. A., Brody, J. I. & Blakemore, W. S., Immunosuppressive effect of surgery. *Lancet* 1, 53 (1971).

45. Klion, F. M., Schaffner, F. & Popper, H., Hepatitis after exposure to halothane. *Ann. Int. Med.* 71, 467 (1969).

46. Uzunalimoglu, B., Yardley, J. H. & Boitnott, J. K., The liver in mild halothane hepatitis. *Amer. J. Path.* 61, 457 (1970).

47. Keeley, A. F., Trey, C., Marcon, N., Iseri, O. A. & Gottlieb, L. S., Anicteric halothane hepatitis: histologic and ultrastructural lesions associated with post-operative fever in two patients. *Gastroenterology* 58, 965 (1970).

48. Babior, B. M. & Davidson, C. S., Post-operative massive livernecrosis. A clinical and pathological study. *New Eng. J. Med.* 276, 645 (1967).

49. Rodriguez, M., Paronetto, F., Schaffner, F. & Popper, H., Antimitochondrial antibodies in jaundice following drug administration *J. Amer. med. Ass.* 208, 148 (1969).

50. Schumer, W., Erve, P. R., Obernolte, R. P., Bombeck, C. T. & Sadove, M. S., The effect of inhalation of halogenated anaesthetics on rat liver mitochondrial function. *Anesthesiology* 35, 253 (1971).
51. Teller, D. N., Denber, H. C. B. & Kopac, M. J., Binding of chlorpromazine and thioproperazine in vitro – 1. *Bioch. Pharm.* 16, 1397 (1967).
52. Sherlock, S., *Diseases of the liver and biliary system.* p. 374. Fourth ed. Oxford 1968.
53. Popper, H., Drug induced liver injury. Read before the New York State Society of Anesthesiologists. New York 1967.
54. Burns, T. H. S., Halothane hepatitis. *Brit. med. J.* 2, 523 (1971).
55. Paronetto, F. & Popper, H., Lymphocyte stimulation induced by halothane in patients with hepatitis following exposure to halothane. *New Eng. J. Med.*, 283, 277 (1970).
56. Doniach, D., Roitt, I. M., Walker, J. G. & Sherlock, S., Tissue antibodies in primary biliary cirrhosis, active chronic (lipoid) hepatitis, cryptogenic cirrhosis and other liver diseases and their clinical implications. *Clin. exp. Immunol.* 1, 237 (1966).
57. Klatskin, G. & Kimberg, D. N., Recurrent hepatitis attributable to halothane sensitisation in an anaesthetist. *New Eng. J. Med.* 280, 515 (1969).
58. *Lancet* 1, 1221 (1971). Management of chronic hepatitis – Leading article.
59. Linde, H. W. & Bruce, D. L., Halothane – occupational exposure. *Anesthesiology* 30, 363 (1969).
60. Hallen, B., Ehrner-Samuel, H. & Thomason, M., Measurements of halothane in the atmosphere of an operating theatre and in expired air and blood of the personnel during routine anaesthetic work. *Acta anaesth. Scand.* 14, 17 (1970).
61. Bruce, D. L., Eide, K. A., Linde, H. W. & Eckenhoff, J. E., Causes of death among anesthesiologists: a 20 year survey. *Anesthesiology* 29, 565 (1968).

THE DANGERS OF ANAESTHETIC AGENTS TO PERSONNEL WORKING IN OPERATING THEATRES

JOH. SPIERDIJK*

During the last few years there has been a growing interest in the working conditions and health of the anaesthetist. The work of the anaesthetist demands constant unimpaired mental alertness and physical fitness. Therefore the working conditions must be optimal.

We are all aware of the difficulties caused by a shortage of anaesthetists. For most of the Dutch anaesthetists it is necessary to work in more than one operating room. Some of us are constantly on call, and this means that it is impossible to get a good rest. In the operating rooms the personnel inhale anaesthetic gases and vapours. This is especially so in the case of anaesthetists who use open, semi-open and non-rebreathing systems. They are constantly inhaling anaesthetic gases: nitrous oxide, halothane or methoxyflurane.

Little is known about the influence of emotional stress upon the anaesthetist during his work. Also we know little about the differences in mental and physical conditions of anaesthetists, surgeons and nurses working in operating theatres. We would like to know the daily state of health of the anaesthetist acting on his ability to detect and to deal with difficult situations influenced by:

Alertness and workload (stress)
Acute poisoning
Chronic poisoning
Combination of the other factors

With the help of the department of psychology (Miss R. Horstink) and Dr. V. Rejger of the anaesthetic department, we attempted to assess the anaesthetist as a member of the surgical team. Does the difference in status of nurses, anaesthetists and surgeons result in mental difficulties amongst the

---

* in conjunction with V. Rejger and Miss J. J. H. van Meeverden.

anaesthetists? These investigations are under progress at the present time, and the different groups of operating personnel are being assessed by psycho-mimetic tests and tests on reaction time to try to look for differences. To study the effects of poisoning two studies were carried out. Firstly, Dutch anaesthetists were asked about working conditions and the state of their health. Secondly, by means of blood tests, the state of health of six anaesthetists was followed after arriving back from their holidays.

Most of the investigations concerning the health of anaesthetists have been done by retrospective studies (1, 2, 3). Bruce et al. investigated the cause of death amongst anaesthetists in the U.S.A. and compared this group with a group of policy holders of an insurance company, and also with U.S. males. The death rate from suicide amongst anaesthetists appeared to be more than twice that of a comparable social economic group of the general population. The incidence of death from malignancies affecting lymphoid and reticuloendothelial tissues appears to be appreciably higher amongst anaesthetists than amongst the general population. The cause of this high death rate from lymphoid and R.E.S. malignancy is unknown. It could be due to radiation, but the data obtained by Bruce et al. (1) as well as that obtained by us, does not confirm this hypothesis (see later). The chronic exposure to volatile anaesthetics, or something not yet identified must play a role!

In 1956 Lassen et al. (4) showed that the prolonged administration of nitrous oxide can give rise to severe depression of the bone marrow. Eastwood and co-workers (5) reported the depression of white cell formation in the albino rat as well as in cases of myelogenous leukaemia. Johnston, Swartz and Donati (6) described erythropoetic and leukopoetic depression occurring in rats during exposure to 80% nitrous oxide. The possibility that the continuous inhalation of anaesthetic vapour can lead to teratogenic or embryocidal effects in man, is still questionable. Smith (7) pointed out that the teratogenic effect of most of the inhalation anaesthetic agents has now been convincingly demonstrated in laboratory animals.

Bruce and Koepke (8) exposed rats continuously for 24-115 hours to 0.45% (4500 p.p.m.) halothane in air. This resulted in the appearance of granulocytic cells in peripheral blood. They suggested that an alteration in cytoplasmic structure and function may be responsible for the inhibition of cellular division. In a latter experiment they exposed rats over an eight month period, for seven hours a day, five days a week, to an environment of 100 part per million halothane in air (1 p.p.m. = 0.0001 vol. %). Compared with a control group no differences were found apart from the fact that the spleens of the exposed rats were heavier. No histological reason for this could be found. Another difference was that the bone marrow in halothane treated rats was slightly more cellular.

Several workers have looked at the concentrations of the anaesthetic in use, at the site of the pop-of value, the presence of air-conditioning in the operating room and measures taken to avoid the accumulation of high concentrations of anaesthetic vapours. The results are summarized in the following table:

| | Anaesthetic vapours in the operating rooms. p.p.m. | | |
	Halothane	N_2O	Meth. Flur.
Corbett-Ball 1			1.3 - 9.8
Corbett-Ball 2*			0.015-0.095
Hallen	Trace - 290		
Linde-Bruce	0 - 49	0 - 354	
Schulze 1	120 - 14200		
Schulze 2*	1000		
Leiden 1968	0.03 - 0.45	2 - 400	
Askrog 1	86	7000	non return
Askrog 2*	9	649	non return

* after venting the vapours.

The venting of vapours from the operating room is necessary to obtain better working conditions. This is made possible by constructing a special valve (3) – a special balloon around the expiratory valve – with a corrugated tube leading to a central vacuum or to the outlet of the air-conditioning system (9, 10). In our department the same modification has been made to an Engstrom ventilator by P. J. Janssen. Schulze (11) constructed a special filter in order to absorb anaesthetic gases – especially halothane by carbon absorbers. The duration of exposure to the anaesthetic vapours, as well as the concentration is also important. Therefore it is necessary to measure the concentration of anaesthetic gases in the anaesthetist. Hallen et al. (12) found that the end expired air of anaesthetists one hour after operation contained up to 300 p.p.m. halothane. In the venous blood they found between 0.021 and 0.63 p.p.m. (In blood 1 p.p.m. halothane = 0.187 mg/%). Linde and Bruce (13) detected 0-12.2 p.p.m. halothane in the end expired air of anaesthetists during or soon after anaesthesia.

Halothane and nitrous oxide are not the only source of risk to the anaesthetist, methoxyflurane must also be considered. Corbett and Ball (10) discovered between 0.1-0.6 p.p.m. of methoxyflurane in the end expired air of anaesthetists 30 hours after operation. Also they found a five-fold increase of the fluoride content of the urine of an anaesthetist, six hours after exposure to methoxyflurane for 390 minutes, under normal working conditions.

Of interest are the findings concerning the genital system. Vaisman (2) reported only seven uneventful pregnancies occurring out of a total of 31. Askrog (3) reported an increase in the incidence of abortion occurring amongst the wives of male anaesthetists, female anaesthetists and nurse-anaesthetists. The total frequency of abortions occurring in Askrog's study are 10% before employment and 20% during employment. His question-naire included 580 nurse-anaesthetists, and 174 female and male anaesthe-tists. All groups of investigated people showed a change in sex ratio, with a reduction in the number of male deliveries. This change was only significant during the first years of employment.

Fink (14) exposed pregnant rats to an atmosphere containing 50% N_2O over 20 days. There was a marked preponderance of destruction of male foetuses resulting in a higher incidence of female deliveries.

As the results of the prospective study are not available, retrospective information concerning the state of health of Dutch anaesthetists is given. Since 1948 the cause of death amongst this group is presented below.

Dutch anaesthetists (1948 n = 13, 1970 n = 284)

Cause of death	Male	Female
RES*	2	1
Myocardial infarction	7	
Malignant disease	1	
Total	10	1

* In the same age group in the Netherlands, six men died from a disease of the reticulo endothelial system, out of a population of 1,055,248 during 1969.

Secondly a questionnaire was sent to 284 members of the Dutch Society of Anaesthetists.

	Total	Male	Female
Members	284	221	63
Replies	123	100	23

Special attention was drawn to the effect on the genital system.

The following answers were obtained:

Female anaesthetists   23

			Not voluntary	Voluntary
Married	with children	5		
	without children	7	5*	2
Not married		11		

* in two cases – known tuberculous infections.

Married female anaesthetists with children

		After starting anaesthetic work
Boys	5	4
Girls	6	3
Extra-uterine		1
Abortions		4

The number of answers submitted by the female anaesthetists is too low for any conclusion to be drawn. It is interesting to look at the offspring of male anaesthetists:

Male anaesthetists   100

Total number of children	Before starting anaesthetic work	After starting anaesthetic work
Boys	67	73
Girls	39	76

Normally the incidence is 100:104/105 – girls:boys.
This data can be analysed by further division:

Male anaesthetists   23

	Before starting anaesthetic work	After starting anaesthetic work
Boys 28	—
Girls 25	—

Male anaesthetists   31

	Before starting anaesthetic work	After starting anaesthetic work
Boys —	32
Girls —	50

Male anaesthetists   34

	Before starting anaesthetic work	After starting anaesthetic work
Boys 41	40
Girls 23	29

If a man starts his family after becoming an anaesthetist he produces more female infants.

The following tables give an impression of some of the other results of the questionnaire.

Male   100

Nervousness		
Sleeping disorders	}	61 (15 with extra systoles)
Irritability		
Disturbance of concentration	5	
Skin reactions	7	
Peptic ulcer	2	
Myocardial infarction	2	
Hypertension	2	

Female   23

Nervousness		
Sleeping disorders	}	14 (4 with extra systoles)
Irritability		
Skin reactions	1	

Also included was a question about the possible relationship between work load and accidents, or between the influence of anaesthetic gases and accidents.

Car accidents after work

	Possible cause	Work load	Halothane
Female	23	1	–
Male	100	14	1

From this it would appear that female anaesthetists are better drivers than their male counterparts.

LIVER

Nine anaesthetists reported the occurrence of a liver disease during anaesthetic work. From eight all the relevant information was collected and no direct influence of anaesthetic agents could be detected. In the literature there are two cases described of hypersensitivity reactions to halothane occurring in anaesthetics.

Apart from the direct effect of anaesthetic gases, there are other factors which may play an important part.

These causes are:

1. Radiation, in the case of malignant disease.
2. Infection – with australia virus in the case of liver disturbance.

RADIATION

Attention is drawn to the teratogenic effect of radiation. All members of the anaesthetic department here in Leiden wore a badge for three months (Radiology Department T.N.O. Institute). The amount of exposure to radiation was measured every 14 days, the smallest measurable amount being 0.02 Rö. The results are presented in the next table.

Department of Anaesthesia, University of Leiden. Members 22. Period: 14 days: maximum exposure allowed 0-2R.

Results:	0.02R	113
	0.03R	1

The highest exposure reported by Linde and Bruce (13) was 95 milliroentgens a week. The results of Askrog and Peterson (15) showed an average of 1.5 MR.

INFECTION

Recently, attention has been drawn to the possibility of the australia antigen being a causal factor in some cases of liver disturbance. In patients with hepatitis a specific acute-phase antigen may be demonstrated (16, 17). This antigen, or its antibodies have been detected in the blood of blood donors and personnel working in laboratories and dialysis centres. Because this antigen was just detected in an Australian aborigine (Blumberg) this antigen has become known as 'australia antigen'. This virus is detected in patients with infections as well as serum hepatitis, so Gocke and Kavey talk about 'hepatitis antigen'.

In New York this virus has been found in 8 out of 1726 apparently healthy donors. In Holland 2 out of 3000 donors in Utrecht and 1 out of 1000 in Amsterdam were positive. The antigen was not detectable in the blood of 20 doctors from the department here, nor, at this date in the blood of the eight anaesthetists with a liver disease in the history, however, during his illness, in the blood of one of the eight, the antigen was detectable.

The history of the only affected anaesthetist here in Leiden is as follows.

A few days after starting work in this department one of the anaesthetists felt sick and tired. His eyes became yellow and his serum bilirubin was found to be 12.04 units, and SGPT 503, SGOT 368. The tests for the australian antigen were positive, and have remained so, even after total recovery.

Oral contamination from the sputum of a patient is possible, as well as by contamination via a skin lesion, through the anaesthetist's fingers entering the mouth of the patient. As a preventative measure it is recommended that a mask should be worn during intubation and suction. Also it is necessary to wear gloves in these circumstances. Since contamination from both donor and patients' blood is possible, it is necessary to be very careful during intravenous injections and the changing of blood bottles.

CONCLUSION

The anaesthetist during his work is influenced by both stress and by low concentrations of anaesthetic gases. Both of these can influence his state of health. The large number of 'nervous' anaesthetists, suffering from extrasystoles can probably be explained by a combination of these factors. The irregular eating habits of the anaesthetist coupled with a high intake of coffee and tea, can also result in extrasystoles. Looking at the direct influence of anaesthetic gases, the information of Bruce must be considered, as well as the above mentioned data about malignant disease of the R.E.S. Radiation appears to have no influence. Health control of anaesthetists is necessary!

This work did not confirm the work of Askrog and Vaisman concerning the incidence of abortion, although from this questionnaire it appeared that more girls are born after starting work with anaesthetic agents. Further investigations are necessary in this field.

Until now we could not detect any influence of anaesthetic gases on liver function. As Professor Simpson mentioned, in the literature, two anaesthetists have been reported to be sensitive to halothane, resulting in hepatitis. However, in the blood of one of the anaesthetists here, and a second anesthetist in the enquiry, the australian virus was found. It would seem necessary that the anaesthetist is made aware of the risk of contamination with blood or oro-pharyngial secretions.

The venting, or absorption of anaesthetic gases from the operating room is strongly recommended, especially when non-rebreathing systems are used.

138 JOH. SPIERDIJK

We agree with Corbett and Ball, that effective exhaust systems should become
standard equipment on all new machines, and devices for adapting existing
machines should be made available as soon as possible. Particular care must
be taken to protect pregnant anaesthetists.

REFERENCES

1. Bruce, D. L., Eide, K. A., Linde, H. W. & Eckenhoff, J. E., Causes of death among
   anesthesiologists; a 20-year survey. *Anesthesiology* 29, 3, 565 (1968).
2. Vaisman, A. I., Working conditions in surgery and their effect on the health of
   anesthesiologists. *Eksp. Khir.* 3, 44 (1967).
3. Askrog, V. F., Dangers of profession. Paper red on the 3rd European Congress of Anaesthesia. Praha 1970.
3a. Askrog, V. F., Eksspirationsventil med udluftningskanal. *Saertryk fra Nordisk Medicin*
   83, 811 (1970).
3b. Askrog, V. F. & Harvald, B., Teratogen effekt af inhalationsanaestetika. *Saertryk fra
   Nordisk Medicin* 83, 498 (1970).
4. Lassen, H. C. A., Henriksen, E., Neukirch, F. & Kristensen, H. S., Treatment of
   tetanus; severe bone-marrow depression after prolonged nitrous-oxide anaesthesia.
   Lancet 527 (1956).
5. Eastwood, D. W., Green, C. D., Lambdin, M. A. & Gardner, R., Effect of nitrous-
   oxide on the white-cell count in leukemia. *New Engl. J. Med.* 268, 6, 297 (1963).
6. Johnson, M. S., Swartz, H. M. & Donati, R. M., Hematologic alterations produced by
   nitrous-oxide. *Anesthesiology* 34, 1, 42 (1971).
7. Smith, B. E., Teratogenicity of inhalation anaesthetics. *Proceedings 4th World Congress of Anesthesiologists.* p. 319 Amsterdam 1970.
8. Bruce, D. L. & Koepke, J. A., Changes in granulopoiesis in the rat associated with
   prolonged halothane anesthesia. *Anesthesiology* 27, 6, 811 (1966).
9. Guitton, M., Les anesthésiques volatils et la santé de l'anesthésiste. *Cah. Anesth.* 19, 1
   (1971).
10. Corbett, T. H. & Ball, G. L., Chronic exposure to methoxyflurane: A possible occupational hazard to anesthesiologists. *Anesthesiology* 34, 6, 532 (1971).
11. Schulze, H. H., Kästner, D. & Lange, P., Zur Frage der chronischen Toxicität von
   Halothankonzentrationen in der Operationssaalluft. *Anaesthesist* 18, 11, 378 (1969).
12. Hallen, B., Ehrner-Samuel, H. & Thomason, M., Measurements of halothane in the
   atmosphere of an operating theatre and in expired air and blood of the personnel during
   routine anesthetic work. *Acta anesth. scand.* 14, 17 (1970).
13. Linde, H. W. & Bruce, D. L., Occupational exposure of anesthetists to halothane,
   nitrous-oxide and radiation. *Anesthesiology* 30, 4, 363 (1969).
14. Fink, B. R. & Simpson, W. E., Cellular metabolic depression by volatile, barbiturate
   and local anesthetics. *Proceedings 4th World Congress of Anesthesiologists* p. 309
   Amsterdam 1970.
15. Askrog, V. & Petersen, R., Forurening af operationsstuer med luftformige anaestetika
   og röntgenbeSträling. *Saertryk fra Nordisk Medicin* 83, 501 (1970).
16. Blumberg, B. S., Alter, H. J. & Visnick, S. A., 'New' antigen in leukemia sera. *J.
   Amer. med. Ass.* 191, 541 (1965).
17. Gocke, D. J. & Kavey, N. B., Hepatitis antigen. Correlation with disease and infec-
   tivity of blood-donors. *Lancet* 1055 (1969).

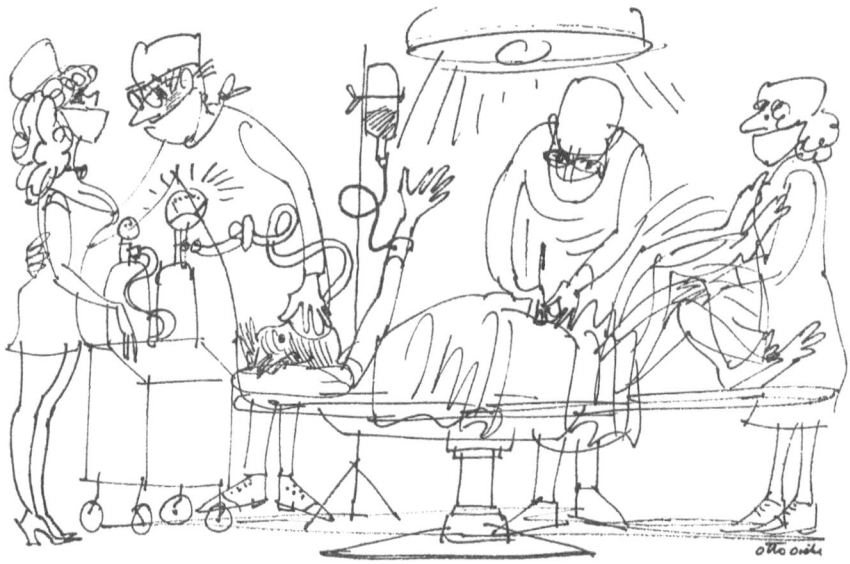

The origin of extrasystoles is sometimes clear!

INDEX OF SUBJECTS

Abbé Fontana 41
Acetazolamide (Diamox)
    prolongation of pentobarbitone action
    by – 109
Acetyl choline 45, 46
Acid-base balance 35
Acid-base changes 64
Acidosis 65, 69, 72, 84, 87
    metabolic – 65, 69, 71
    respiratory – 65, 69, 71
Acetylcholine 49, 51, 52, 54, 55, 56, 57,
    59, 60, 61, 62
Adrenaline 38, 97, 101
Adductor pollicis muscle 67
Affinity 42
    constant – 43, 46
    constant high – 44, 54
    constant low – 45
    high – 44
Air-conditioning 132
Alcuronium 33, 77, 83
    radium active – 77
Alkalosis 65, 72
    hypochloremic – 98
    metabolic – 67, 69, 70
    respiratory – 69, 70, 71
Alpha blockade 101
Alpha-methyldopa 96
Alpha-methylnoradrenaline 96
Amphetamine 97
Anaesthesia
    induction of – 99
Anatomical construction 46
Anephric patients 78, 80, 85, 87
Antagonists
    competitive – 41
Anterior tibalis muscle 67
Antigen 120, 123, 124, 125, 126

Anti-hypertensive therapy 91
Arfonad 95
Arterial-venous anastomoses 7, 9, 10, 11,
    12
ATP 4, 5, 15
Atropine 19, 35, 76, 78, 95
Australia antigen 136, 137

Barbiturate anaesthesia, enhancement by
    Imipramine (Tofranil) 110
Barbiturate intoxication
    effect of pH in treatment 113
Battery 31
Beta – activator 18
    blockade 20
    receptors 97, 101
    stimulant 20
Bernard, Claude 41
Biophase time 43
Biphasic response 54
Block
    alpha – 101
    beta – 20
    duration of – 46
    magnitude of – 46
    Phase I 45, 46
    Phase II 45, 46, 58
Blockers
    alpha – 3, 5, 6, 8, 9, 10, 12, 13, 14, 15,
    16
    beta – 9, 10, 11, 12, 13, 14, 15, 16
Bradycardia 99

Calcium 32, 33, 34
    – shifts 5, 6, 7, 14
Capacitance vessels 94
Capnogram 36
Capnograph 38

141

Capnographic control 34
Carbon absorbers 132
Cardiac
– arrhytmias 98
– output 19, 25, 26
– pacing 30
Cardiogenic shock 18
Catecholamines 4, 5, 15, 34
Cells 80
Central venous pressure 32, 35, 94, 99, 102
Chlorothalidone 98
Chlorotiazide 98
Chlorpromazine 15, 125
enhancement of nitrous oxide effect by – 107
Cholinergic mechanisms 49
Cholinergic receptor
occupying the – 41
Chronotropic 18, 20, 21, 22, 54, 57, 60, 62
Competition 41
Condamine, de la – 41
Contraction
force of – 43
Coumarin anticoagulants
increased breakdown by barbiturates 112
Curare 43, 44, 45
Cyclopropane 77, 78
– cardiac irregularities suppressed by propranolol 107

Decamethonium 44
Diallyl-bis-nortoxiferin 36
Diamox, see acetazolamide 109
Diaphragm 67
Diazepam 31, 35, 76, 78, 85, 87, 99
Digitalis toxicity 98
Dimethyl curare 43
2.3 Diphosphoglyceric acid 26
Diuretics 98
DMO 69
Droperidol 99, 101
Drug metabolizing enzymes 111
Drug-receptor bonds 42
D-tubocurarine 33, 44, 74, 77, 80, 81, 82, 83, 87
– chloride 49, 51, 52
Dysrrhytmias 99

Ectopic 19

Effects
chronotropic – 101
inotropic – 101
Electro
– cardiogram 32
– cardioscope 32
– cautery 38
Electrode 38
intravenous – 31
Embryocidal 131
Ephidrine 97
Ethacrinic acid 98
Ether 82, 83
curariform effect of – 106

Fentanyl 99
Fever
post-operative – 119
Fluoride 133

Gallamine triethiodide 33, 43, 44, 49, 51, 52, 54, 57, 58, 61, 62, 74, 77, 82
Genital system 133
Gentamycin
neuromuscular blockade by – 106
Glycocen phosphorylation 4
Guanethidine 96

Halothane 76, 80, 82, 83, 96, 101, 116, 118, 119, 120, 121, 122, 123, 124, 125, 126
effect of pentobarbitone on breakdown of – 112
hepatitis 116, 119, 120, 123, 124, 125, 126
National Study 117, 120, 122, 124, 125
Heart block 18, 19, 96
Heart
isolated rabbit 48, 56, 57, 62
Hepatic dysfunction 122
Hepatic necrosis 118, 119, 121, 124
Hepatitis 120, 123, 126
viral – 119, 120, 122, 123, 124, 126
Hepatotoxic 117, 123
Hepatotoxin 122, 123
Histamine 33
Humidification 28
Hydergine 15
Hydralaxine 97
Hydrochlorotrazide 98
Hyperbaric oxygenation 27
Hypercapnia 34
Hyperpotassemia 33

Hyperpyrexia 123
Hypersensitivity 124, 125, 126
Hypertension
    borderline – 93
    labile – 93
    moderate – 92
    secondary – 91
    untreated – 92
    untreated essential – 93
Hypertensive
– crisis 97
– patients 99
– patients untreated 100
Hyperventilation 25
Hypocapnia 25
Hypokalaemia 98, 99
Hypoventilation 25, 26
Hypovolemia 32, 96
Hypoxia 34

Imipramine (Tofranil)
    enhancement of barbiturate anaesthesia
    by – 110
Infection 136
Inotropic 18, 19, 20, 21, 22
    negative – 54
Interactions of drugs 104-115
Intubation
    endotracheal – 99
Isoprenaline 18, 19, 20, 21
– infusion 20, 21
Isuprel 38

Jaundice 117, 118, 119, 120, 121, 123, 125

K/Ca balance 36
Kidney transplantation 77

Lactacidemia 13
Laryngoscopy 99
Leukaemia 131
Lignocaine 34, 38
Liver
– damage 116, 117, 118, 121, 122, 123, 124, 125
– disturbance 136
Lymphoid 131

Mephentermine 38, 97
Metaraminol 97
Methamphetamine 97
Methohexitone 99

Methoxamine hydrochloride 97
Methoxyflurane 76, 78, 83, 125
Methyldopa 96
Mitochondria 24
Monoamine oxidase inhibitor 96
Muscle
    adductor pollicis 67
    anterior tibialis 67
    fast and slow 67
    soleus 67
Muscle relaxants 48, 97, 98
    action of – 97
    pharmacodynamics of – 41
Myoneural junction 46

Neomycin, neuromuscular
    blockade by – 106
Neostigmine 84
Nephrectomy bilateral 74, 78
Nerve stimulator 43, 81, 82
Neurolept anaesthesia 76, 78, 82
Neurolept analgesia 15, 83
Neuro muscular transmission 64
Nico-morphine 36
Nitrous oxide 76, 80, 83
    enhancement by chlorpromazine and reserpine 107
Noradrenaline 20, 96, 97, 101
Norepinephrine 20
Nurse-anaesthetist 133

Oxygen 24, 25, 26, 27, 28
– administration 28
    alveolar tension 27
    arterial saturation 25
    arterial tension 25, 27
– concentration 24, 26, 27, 28
– dissocation curve 26
    hyperbaric – 28
– tension 24

Pacemaker 19, 30, 31, 32, 33, 34, 35, 38
Pancuronium 33, 77, 78, 82, 83, 84, 85, 86, 87
– bromide 36, 49, 51, 52, 57, 61, 62
Pargyline 97
Patients digitalised 96
Peak plasma level 44
Pentobarbitone
    prolongation of action by acetazolamide (Diamox) 109
    effect on halothane breakdown 112

Personnel operating-room 126
Pethidine 76
pH, effect of – on drug excretion 113
Phenobarbitone, enhancement of drug
    metabolism by – 111
Phenylepinephrine 20
Phenyleprine 97, 101
Phrenic nerve-diaphragm preparation 67
Plethysmogram 35
Potassium 33, 35, 79, 80, 85
–/calcium balance 33
– chloride 99
– concentration extracellular 73
–   – intracellular 73
– depletion 98
Potentation
    post-tetanic – 45
Practolole 34, 38
Pregnancies 133
Procainamide 34, 38
Promethazine 31, 35, 76
Propanidid 99
Propranolol 8, 15, 16, 97
    suppression of cyclopropane arrhyth-
    mias 107
Protein binding of drugs 110
Pseudocholinesterase 78
Pulmonary oxygen toxicity 27

Quinidine
    recurarisation by – 110

Radiation 131, 136
Rate theory 42
Rauwolfia alkaloids 95, 96
Receptors
    alpha – 20
    beta – 20
Recurarisation 84
– by quinidine 110
Renal insufficiency 74

Renal transplant 75, 78, 79
Reserpine 95, 96, 101
    enhancement of nitrous oxide effect by –
    107
Resistance vessels 94, 97
Respiratory 69
Resting membrane potential 72, 73
Reticuloendothelial 131

Salicylates and hyperventilation 108
Serpasil 95
Serum K/Ca ratio 34, 38
Serum potassium 99
Sino-atrial node 54, 57, 62
SKF 525-A 112
Stimulation 45
Stimuli
    tetanic – 45
Stimulus threshold 31
Succinylcholine 33, 36, 54, 55, 56, 57, 58,
    59, 60, 61, 62, 74, 76, 77, 78, 79, 80, 87
    dual action 57
Suicide 131

Tachycardia 99
Teratogenic 131, 136
Thalamonal 76
Thiopentone 35, 99
Tissues 131
Tissue perfusion 102
Tofranil, see Imipramine 110
Trimetaphan 95
Tyramine 97

Ventricular
    extrasystoles 34
    fibrillation 34
    tachycardia 34
Veratrum alkaloids 94
Viral infection 124
Volume expanders 32